DREAM STORIES:
Unlocking Your Night Parables
by Michael B. French

"*Dream Stories* is powerfully captivating, penetrating, and easy to understand, yet practical and deeply profound. Christ-centered and submitted to the Word, this book is a relevant and valuable resource for learning to hear God and drawing into deeper intimacy with Him."
LeeArthur J. Madison, apostle and senior pastor, Transformation Ministries International, Washington

"*Dream Stories* is yet another fine work by the brilliantly gifted Michael French. Michael's latest work on the topic of dreams will be both useful and inspirational to the reader. His skillful approach has a way of making the mystical approachable and the complicated easy. Anyone interested in dream interpretation will want this book added to their collection."
Tom Zawacki, pastor, Charlottetown Vineyard, Canada

"Michael has done a great service to the Christian community by sharing *Dream Stories* with us. The need to receive and understand what God is saying has never been greater. Opening up the understanding of dreams to the body of Christ is both needed and necessary. I highly recommend this book to every believer who desires to receive and understand what God is saying to them."
Steve Watson, senior pastor, The Bridge Church, Washington

Having scanned the print media and online for acquiring meaningful and biblical content on understanding dreams, visions, and dream interpretation, we hardly came across much content on the subject. After going through Michael's well-balanced *Dream Stories*, my understanding grew much. I endorse and recommend this book to leaders, practitioners, and learners. Michael's great passion and focused vision on the subject has enabled him to accomplish the mission.

Benito Rogtao, pastor, New Life Fellowship/Connect-India, Mumbai, India

"*Dream Stories* is by far one of the most important books about biblical dream interpretation. I personally believe that the world has been waiting to have this—something to give some better and clearer guidelines on the subject. In this book, you can find practical terms and examples that everyone can draw insights from and to dive deep in their personal dream lives with God. I can foresee this book powerfully transforming millions of lives and lead people to encounter the depth of God.

Rose Wenceslao, Director, Streams Asia, Founder, Created4More, Warnbro, Australia

"In *Dream Stories*, Michael French relays the points that he is trying to make to the reader with such clarity, precision, and impact. I also enjoyed that he used relevant and modern-day examples of dreams for his explanations."

James Tan, IT Manager, Innovasia Inc., Hong Kong, China

Visit
www.MyDreamStories.com

Dreams are certainly one of the many ways that God communicates with His people. This book presents over fifty dreams from real people, so that the reader can hear a dream and its interpretation, and then see how it came to pass and affected the dreamer's life—solid proof that dreams really are telling us something. This book also provides background for dream interpretation and a section about famous people and their dreams.

Dream Stories:
Unlocking Your Night Parables
Michael B. French
Copyright @ 2017 ShadeTree Publishing, LLC
Print ISBN: 978-1-937331-72-6
e-Book ISBN: 978-1-937331-73-3

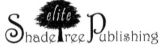

Visit our Web site at www.ShadeTreePublishing.com.

CONTENTS

FOREWORD

by Roxanne Richardson and Chris Mileski, 93.7 WDJC

After many years spent news reporting and witnessing the undisguised deception rampant in our society (sometimes meant purely for monetary gain), WDJC's Roxanne thought the idea of dream interpretation was synonymous with the use of a crystal ball or a psychic friends network. Roxanne's news nose could easily sniff a farce, so when Pastor Michael B. French suggested that he was learning about dream interpretation and was using it as ministry tool, it gave her pause. While she had come a long way from cynicism following her conversion to Christianity, she was still very hesitant to accept what she thought was Michael's "unorthodox" approach to evangelism. And she certainly wasn't in a hurry to submit her Christian radio listeners to such philosophies.

Roxanne began to search the Scriptures for information about dreams. She discovered that if we believe in the Bible, then we clearly see that dreams can mean something, and they can be interpreted. Joseph, the husband of Mary, was visited by an angel in a dream three times. Joseph, the son of Jacob in the Old Testament, interpreted dreams for some fellow prisoners and then for Pharaoh. In Bible times, people knew that their dreams might be from God, and when they didn't understand the spiritual meaning of a dream, they'd seek the help of a discerning prophet of the Lord. Abraham, Jacob, Joseph, Gideon, Peter, Paul, and others all received guidance from God by paying attention to their dreams.

It was Chris who encouraged Roxanne to bring dream interpretation to the radio airwaves. By that time, the pair had spent hours visiting with Michael, getting to appreciate his brilliant mind (he had been trained as an attorney), and great heart (he traveled the world to minister the Gospel). Chris trusted Michael's absolute adherence to listening carefully to the Holy Spirit's promptings, and Roxanne was deeply touched by his honesty—especially when he admitted that he didn't always hear that still, small voice regarding every dream shared with him.

The rest is history. Once Michael appeared as a guest on the radio show, the phone lines were flooded with people who were fascinated to know how God speaks to them through their dreams and what they might mean. Caller after caller expressed gratitude for a deeper understanding of their dreams, especially recurring ones. We long for the discernment of God's wisdom in our lives. Listening to dreams has proven to helpful to our radio listeners, so that they can get back on the right track. God can work through dreams, in part to guide us, or to warn us:

> *In a dream, in a vision of the night, when deep sleep falls on people as they slumber in their beds, he may speak in their ears and terrify them with warnings, to turn them from wrongdoing and keep them from pride, to preserve them from the pit, their lives from perishing by the sword.* —Job 33:15–18 (NIV)

Dream Stories: Learning from God's Night Parables is Michael's labor of love for the Lord, comprised in part by our radio listeners' dreams, shared publicly with the hope that a deeper understanding of them might be gained. It honors the dreamer by providing his or her understanding and interpretation of the dream. It also points to the fact that God is not the source of all of our dreams. As Michael states, "Some dreams are intended to steer the dreamer away from God." That makes this book all the more important—and relevant, too, for as Michael also says, "We live in a world that's almost forgotten the beauty of dreams."

About Roxanne and Chris

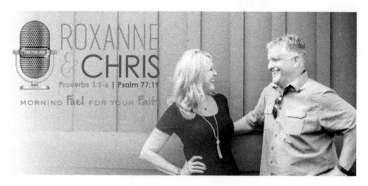

Lisa "Roxanne" Richardson and Chris Mileski are the morning show hosts on Alabama's largest Christian radio station, WDJC FM 93.7. Roxanne and Chris energize the morning airwaves by sharing the power of God's grace and hope in a way that is real and relevant in today's uncertain world. Through listening in to the best in Christian music, storytelling, and special guests, you will find yourself fired up and equipped for the day ahead. Promising plenty of laughs and an occasional tear, this show won't just start your morning—it will fuel your faith to walk in your purpose all day long.

INTRODUCTION

A young woman dreams of planes crashing into two tall towers days just before the events of September 11, 2001. A soldier sees the placement of enemy land mines in a dream and saves the lives of hundreds in Korea. A Muslim is introduced to Christianity by a man dressed in radiant white who visits him in a dream. An inventor dreams that he is about to be executed by savages whose spears have holes in their tips, and he awakens to change the textile industry forever. A young man learns the identity of his biological father from the events he experiences in several dreams. These are "Dream Stories"—testimonies of lives changed by revelation that came from dreams sent by God.

If a picture is worth a thousand words, then a dream filled with images is certainly worth ten thousand. A parable is a simple story (like the ones told by Jesus in the New Testament) to illustrate a moral or a spiritual lesson. If we truly believe that God is still speaking to His people today, then it might be valuable for us to begin thinking of our dreams as night parables from God. After all, dreams are like mini-movies, conveying stories to our spirits.

Dreams and visions occupy a large part of the Scriptures. From Daniel and Joseph in the Old Testament, to Joseph (Mary's husband), Pilate's wife, John (the beloved disciple), and more in the New Testament, dreams and visions have helped God's people to hear His voice. Dreams themselves can be revelatory or prophetic in their nature—that is, they can involve both the concept of foretelling and that of forth-telling. Some dreams, such as those Daniel had, foretell what will happen. Other dreams, such as those Pilot's wife had, can proclaim news or truths. In either case, dreams may be classified—in a biblical sense—as a type of prophecy. This understanding helps us to overcome one of the primary modern objections to dreams and dream interpretation, as veering too far from the message of Jesus. Revelation 19:10 is clear on this point as it declares, "...the testimony of Jesus is the spirit of prophecy" (ESV).

Dreams and biblical dream interpretation are certainly one of many ways that God has chosen to communicate with His people. For those who take a cessationist perspective on theological matters (i.e., believing that spiritual gifts ceased after the apostolic age), this book is not intended to justify the continued existence of the gifts given by the Holy Spirit. Instead, it is the intention of this book to explore the biblical validity of dreams as a means of communication from God, and to help the reader understand their value. Neither is this book intended to provide an in-depth understanding on how to interpret dreams, nor does it provide a "dictionary" of metaphors found in dreams. Rather, it is designed to help the reader gain insight into the validity of dreams as a spiritual encounter, and recognize the impact that dreams can have on the lives of believers and unbelievers alike. To that end and for those who believe that God continues to speak to His people, this book is filled with wonderful illustrations of how dreams have changed lives, as well as explanations of why they are a very real source of inspiration in a world that has almost forgotten the beauty of dreams and the magnitude of their Giver's unfathomable character in using them to continue telling His story.

PART 1
THE VALUE OF DREAMS

The first part of this book is intended to provide you with a basic understanding of biblical dream interpretation and its value for our contemporary culture. While it is difficult to deny the significance of dreams as found in the Scriptures, the value of dreams in a modern context can and has been questioned. Such questioning is only fair, since much of what has been passed off as dream interpretation in Western culture over the past several decades has really been psychological experimentation or New Age religious ideology.

If the Church is truly going to recognize that dreams and biblical dream interpretation are significant, then the foundational elements of Part 1 must be understood. Before we can find it within ourselves to learn from our own dreams, and certainly before we could begin to learn from the dreams of others, we must accept that God speaks and that at times He speaks through dreams. The first part of this book is not intended to convince you of this truth, but rather to provide you with the resources to become a Berean (Acts 17:11) and to seek out the reality of that truth for yourself.

Once you have found the value in dreams, you should be able to see the value in a specific dream, whether it be yours or another's. Keep in mind that it is not really the dream itself that is valuable, but rather it is the God who gives the dream and the increase in relationship that comes from hearing Him. My hope as I write this book is not ultimately to help you find more significance in the dreams you have, but truly to help you draw closer to the Giver of those dreams. After all, it is not the gift that counts, but rather the Giver of the gift. You should never value dreams unless they lead you to place even greater value on the One who speaks to you through them.

The Foundation of Dreams and Biblical Dream Interpretation

While our Western culture tends to devalue dreams, people of the ancient Near East (and even the modern Near East) have always placed a high value upon them. Traditionally, dreams have almost always been viewed as being a form of communication from a deity. The Hebrew people were among those throughout the centuries who have valued dreams and who believed that God (Yahweh) spoke into the lives of His creation through them. Some scholars trace the decline in the valuation of dreams to Aristotle, an ancient Greek philosopher, who maintained that anything that is not tangible is irrelevant. One of Aristotle's main focuses was the systematic concept of logic; according to this way of thinking, only that which had substance was real, and spiritual things were thereby unknowable—basically, if you cannot see it, hear it, smell it, taste it, or feel it, then it has no value. This Greek mindset, rather than the Hebrew one, has prevailed in our Western culture.

Many Hebrews believed that if someone went a week without a significant dream, then God was unhappy with them. This thought carried on into early Judeo-Christian philosophy. While it may not follow that God is unhappy with us when we do not remember our dreams, this belief clearly indicates the importance placed on dreams in the early days of our own Christian faith. Lest anyone think that such historical and philosophical rationale for accepting the significance of dreams is lacking in a biblical foundation, keep in mind that God Himself emphasized the importance of dreams as one of the ways in which He speaks:

> *And he said, "Hear my words: If there is a prophet among you, I the Lord make myself known to him in a vision; I speak with him in a dream.* —Numbers 12:6 (ESV)

This reference to dreams in the Scriptures is only one among many. Jeremiah warned God's people to be careful of those who used dreams to prophesy falsely (Jeremiah 23:32). While this may seem to be more of a warning concerning dreams, consider the fact that there would be no need to warn people of something that could be abused, if there were no true prophetic dreams in the first place.

With Jeremiah's warning in mind, some scholars have argued that dreams should not be taken into consideration as a means of communication from God, due to the risk that they could easily be counterfeited or tainted. Yet the possibility of counterfeit or tainted dreams is not a valid excuse for rejecting them altogether. Think about this argument as you consider the following analogy.

The twenty-dollar bill is one of the most widely distributed pieces of currency not only in the United States, but also throughout the world. In fact, the odds favor the likelihood of those reading these words actually having a twenty-dollar bill in their possession as they read. Yet, according to records kept by the United States Treasury Department, the United States Secret Service, and the Federal Reserve, the twenty-dollar bill is among the most frequently encountered counterfeit bills in the world (with only the one-hundred-dollar bill surpassing it in terms of value of the currency counterfeited). In addition, according to a story reported in 2009 by CNN, "Research presented...reinforced previous findings that ninety percent of paper money circulating in U.S. cities contains traces of cocaine."[1] Despite these undeniable statistics, it is highly unlikely that people reading this are going to now throw out their twenty-dollar bill and refuse to use it.

If we are unwilling to give up our twenty-dollar bills despite the overwhelming odds that they are either counterfeit or tainted by traces of drugs, yet we refuse to consider dreams as a possible means of communication with God because they may be false or corrupted, then there are more pressing concerns about the state of our spirituality than can be addressed by the scope of this book.

The Bible is filled with dreams that changed the lives of individuals and the course of nations. Without attempting an exhaustive and detailed recounting of every dream in the Scriptures the following list should provide ample evidence that the men and women of the Bible overcame any fears regarding the potential for false or tainted dreams and they embraced this amazing way in which God communicates:

Abraham and Israel's Coming Captivity (Genesis 15:12–21). The patriarch Abraham (actually, at that time he was still known as Abram) was told of Israel's coming captivity during a visitation that occurred while he was in a deep sleep. This dream conveyed God's promise and encouraged Abraham to believe for what he could not yet see.

Abimelech's Warning Not to Take Sarah (Genesis 20:3). Only a short time after

Abraham's dream encounter, the first dream was given to communicate with a non-believer as God told Abimelech not to go in to Abraham's wife, Sarah. This was a warning dream both to protect Abimelech from the judgment of God, and to protect Abraham and Sarah from the consequences of their actions.

Jacob's Ladder (Genesis 28:11–19). This encounter with the angels ascending and descending that famous ladder occurred at a place called Bethel during a dream. By giving this dream to Jacob, God not only encouraged him, but He began a work of transformation in his life.

Jacob and His Increase in Wealth (Genesis 31:10–13). Jacob was instructed in a dream to go against tradition and take the spotted and speckled of his father-in-law's flocks. Courage was imparted to Jacob by this dream, allowing him to go against his cultures understanding of animal husbandry and to obtain provision that could only have come from God.

Laban's Warning (Genesis 31:29). God spoke to Laban in the night, warning him not to stand against Jacob. This warning dream not only preserved Jacob's safety, but it also preserved family relationships that might otherwise have stayed broken forever.

Joseph's Dreams of Sheaves and Stars (Genesis 37:5–11). Actually, in two separate dreams, Joseph learned of his destiny. Joseph would later go through the experiences of the pit and the prison, during which time he would need the encouragement of God's promise in order to endure.

The Cupbearer's Dream (Genesis 40:1–13). While in prison, Joseph interpreted this dream of restoration. This dream and the next one were both for the benefit of the dreamer and the interpreter. Joseph would be remembered as an interpreter of dreams. The butler, on the other hand, had both the opportunity to encounter God and to be encouraged by His all-knowing nature.

The Baker's Dream (Genesis 40:16–22). Unlike the cupbearer, the baker received an unpleasant interpretation to his dream. Though the interpretation might have been unpleasant, the revelation of it gave this dreamer the opportunity to prepare for what what was about to come.

Pharaoh's Dreams of Cows and Grain (Genesis 41:15–44). These two dreams by the world's most powerful ruler elevated Joseph to a position of prominence and preserved not only a single nation, but also much of the world, from starvation. These dreams not only preserved a nation (and, some might say, the known world), their interpretation by Joseph established him in the position of destiny that God had promised in his own dreams years before.

Gideon's Encouragement (Judges 7:13–15). This dream was not actually experienced by

Gideon, but when the Midianite soldier recounted the experience, it was Gideon who began to worship. God used this dream to confirm that it was He who would defeat the Midianites and to place courage into the heart of Gideon as he heard it shared.

Solomon's Wisdom (1 Kings 3:5–15). This famous question-and-answer session resulting in more than Solomon could ask or imagine, took place in a dream. This was both a dream and an encounter with God through that dream. It provided a means by which God and Solomon could interact directly.

Nebuchadnezzar and Daniel (Daniel 2). In this encounter, God not only revealed the interpretation of Nebuchadnezzar's dream to Daniel, but He also gave the dream itself. By giving Daniel both the dream and the interpretation, God established that it was He alone (not even Danial) who knew the hearts of men.

Nebuchadnezzar's Second Dream (Daniel 4). This dream of a great tree is a call to repentance also interpreted by Daniel. Nebuchadnezzar's heart was revealed and ultimately changed by this dream.

Daniel's Dream (Daniel 7). Not only is Daniel a gifted interpreter of dreams, he is also a dreamer. This is a prophetic dream/vision, the full understanding of which remains veiled.

Joseph's Dream (Matthew 1:20–21). Through a dream, Joseph was encouraged to take Mary as his wife, despite her virgin conception. The courage imparted by this dream allowed Joseph to overcome the cultural stigmas that would have resulted from taking the pregnant Mary as his wife.

The Wise Men's Dream (Matthew 2:12). The Magi were warned not to return to Herod through a dream. God chose a dream as the means to communicate this message that would literally preserve the life of the Messiah.

Joseph's Second Dream (Matthew 2:13). Mary and Joseph's flight to Egypt was the result of a dream. Once again, this was a dream that preserved Jesus' life.

Joseph's Third Dream (Matthew 2:19–21). The instructions for Mary and Joseph to return to Israel also come in a dream. This dream was less about protection and more about timing, providing Joseph and Mary with the insight that they could now return home.

Joseph's Fourth Dream (Matthew 2:22–23). This dream warning to Joseph sends him and his family to the district of Galilee and the city of Nazareth. This was a directional dream that provided information about the geographical location where Jesus should be raised, thus fulfilling several Messianic prophecies from the Old Testament.

Pilate's Wife's Dreams (Matthew 27:19). Another nonbeliever whose dream established the innocence of Jesus. Though we know little about the details of this dream, it is perhaps one of the most significant dreams in the Scriptures. This dream resulted in a public declaration before the man who held Jesus' life in his hand, and that innocent blood would be shed if Christ were crucified.

The Relationship Between Dreams and Visions

For many people, the difference between a dream and a vision is that the former occurs during the night while we are sleeping, and the latter occurs during the daytime while we are awake. This distinction, of course, may hold true in many instances, but it is not sufficient when it comes to helping us establish a foundation through which we can begin to understand and value dreams. Lest anyone feel alone in their confusion over this matter, the relationship between and difficulty in distinguishing dreams and visions is long-standing.

There are approximately two hundred references to dreams or visions in the Scriptures, and as much as one third of the Scriptures relate either directly or indirectly to a dream or a vision. With this many references to dreams and visions, it is not surprising that we would find that the Bible characters also had some difficulty in establishing the appropriate terminology for which is which. Consider the somewhat confusing language used in the book of Daniel and elsewhere when it comes to this topic: "in a dream, in a vision of the night" in Job 33:15 (NIV); "your dream and the visions of your head as you lay in bed" in Daniel 2:28 (ESV); "visions of my dream" in Daniel 4:9 (ESV); "a dream, a vision of the night" in Daniel 7:1, and "dream of a night vision" in Isaiah 29:7 (ESV).

With such diverse use of terminology, it seems important to have a consistent understanding of the distinction between dreams and visions, if only for the purpose of clarity in this book. With that in mind, what is the difference between a dream and a vision? A dream is not merely a mini-movie that occurs only while we are asleep. Instead, it should be considered a spiritual encounter in which most, if not all, of the images seen are metaphoric and symbolic in nature and therefore in need of interpretation. On the other hand, a vision is not limited to a mini-movie that plays out while we are awake. Instead, it should be considered a spiritual encounter in which most, if not all, of the images seen are more literal and thereby requiring very limited interpretation, if any. These definitions, while certainly not definitive, allow us to stay much more consistent with the language of Job, Daniel, and Isaiah. There certainly may be elements of dreams that do not need interpretation and elements of visions that do, but for the simplest distinction between dreams and visions, it is better to consider dreams as needing interpretation whereas visions are more literal, than it is to assume that they take place only at night.

Dreams, being both a means of God's communicating with His people and a mystery that must be unraveled, can be seen as an enigma that draws the creation closer to the Creator. Proverbs 25:2 declares that, "It is the glory of God to conceal things, but the glory of kings is to search things out" (ESV). We, as kings and priests, are charged with the task of searching out the things that God conceals, and what He conceals in the dreams that He gives us can be well worth the effort associated with the search. Many people desire God to speak the clearest and the loudest during our times of greatest difficulty, yet it is often more common for these to be the times when He speaks the most quietly. In the very moments when we are longing for God to shout, He chooses to whisper. We can keep our distance and still hear the instructions contained in the shout, but when we want to understand what is communicated in the whisper, we must draw intimately close to the One doing the whispering. In this manner, we should consider dreams to be God's whispering call to our spirit man. If the mystery of a dream is not drawing us closer to the God who gives it, then, despite the message contained therein, it is of little value. On the other hand, when a dream calls us closer, it can be a very present help in time of trouble (see Psalm 46:1).

Sources of Our Dreams

The idea of God whispering secrets to us while we sleep is a beautiful concept, but it does not account for those dreams at the opposite end of the spectrum, the ones that terrify us. This, then, raises the question of where our dreams come from. Is God the Source of all of our dreams?

Dreams can originate from at least three different sources, and therefore God is not the author of all of them. Since the early days of Church history, at least as early as the time of Tertullian's writings, dreams have been seen as originating either with God, with the enemy, or from within our own soul. The greatest value and primary focus of this book is, of course, those dreams that come from God. However, it is certainly important to provide a minimal examination of the other two sources for our dreams.

Without question, dreams from God should be a source of joy and encouragement in the life of the dreamer. However, when they are properly understood, dreams from the enemy and dreams produced by our own soul can also become a source of joy and encouragement. Though the dream itself may not be encouraging, dreams from these two secondary sources that are interpreted with the wisdom of the Holy Spirit will often provide insight into how God sees the situation that goes beyond their base meaning. Keep in mind that when a Spirit-led interpretation is given to any dream, it is a good and valuable dream.

Some dreams are intended to steer the dreamer away from God and into places of darkness. The source of these dreams has to be considered demonic, and Jeremiah warns us of those dreams:

> *Behold, I am against those who prophesy lying dreams, declares the Lord, and who tell them and lead my people astray by their lies and their recklessness, when I did not send them or charge them. So they do not profit this people at all, declares the Lord.* —Jeremiah 23:32 (ESV)

Jeremiah goes on to establish clearly that such "false dreams" should not be heeded as they are lies and "[God] did not send them" (Jeremiah 29:8–9 ESV). These dreams, as well as nightmares, fear dreams, and in most cases, spiritual warfare dreams, originate not with God, but instead with our adversary, the devil, who is the father of lies according to John 8:44.

While there is little redemptive value in false prophetic dreams sent by the enemy to deceive and lead people astray (or as Zechariah puts it, cause "the people [to] wander like sheep [that] are afflicted for lack of a shepherd" [Zechariah 10:2, ESV], God-sent understanding of such dreams can at least reveal the plan of the enemy and encourage those who are willing to stand against such plans. One of the greatest dream interpreters of all time, Joseph, understood this basic principle when he declared in Genesis 50:20, "As for you, you meant evil against me, but God meant it for good . . ." (ESV). If we trust Him, God will not allow even such dark dreams to be wasted, but He will use them to bring about good despite the plans of the enemy to the contrary.

The first two sources of our dreams (God and the devil) are external in their nature; however, the final source can be viewed as much more internal—our own soul. This source tends to involve the recitation in our dreams of the longings and desires put forth by our own mind, will, and emotions. Such dreams tend to convey much more information about the dreamer's own thoughts and feelings and should not be viewed as communication from God. Consider Solomon's wisdom from the book of Ecclesiastes as one explanation of such dreams:

> *A dream comes when there are many cares,*
> *and many words mark the speech of a fool.* —
> Ecclesiastes 5:3 (NIV)

As Solomon understood it, there are times when the cares of life weigh heavily upon us, and it is these matters that work their way into our dream life. While the anxieties of life contribute to this soulish source of dreams, the personal desires of the dreamer can also be a factor:

> *As when a hungry man dreams he is eating*
> *and awakes with his hunger not satisfied, or*
> *as when a thirsty man dreams he is drinking*
> *and awakes faint, with his thirst not*
> *quenched, so shall the multitude of all the*
> *nations be that fight against Mount Zion.* —
> Isaiah 29:8 (ESV)

Isaiah went on to explain that the love of sleep, even among those who have no spiritual insight whatsoever, can result in dreams that do not trace their origin back to either God or the devil (Isaiah 56:10).

Sources of Dream Interpretation

If our dreams themselves can originate from multiple sources and it is essential for us to look to God as the Source of our interpretation in order to redeem those dreams that do not originate with Him, then it should not be surprising that our adversary would also establish false methods of interpretation in his efforts to discredit this source of revelation. Those who fear counterfeit dreams will frequently point to this topic as yet another reason why dreams and dream interpretation should be avoided. But for those who choose to keep their twenty-dollar bills and their dreams as a source of wealth, this risk does not rise to a level that requires abstinence. When a banker is taught to recognize a counterfeit twenty-dollar bill, no great amount of time is spent in the examination of all the possible ways it can be counterfeited. This is true because there are hundreds if not thousands of minute variations in the way a bill can be counterfeited. Instead, the focus of anti-counterfeit education is placed upon knowing the real thing, with an understanding that if one has an intimate knowledge of the real thing, then the counterfeit will be easily identified. With that concept in mind, only a cursory examination of the false means of interpretation is necessary here.

Suffice it to say that the primary sources of dream interpretation parallel the sources of our dreams. Interpretation can also come from God, the enemy, or our own soul. However, it should be noted that in the case of interpretation, if it does not come from God, it matters little whether the source is directly from some non-Christian spiritual mechanism or a product of own soulish efforts, because our adversary is actively behind either means. New Age or Eastern religious means of interpretation (as well as other false religious methods) are often readily identifiable, as those who use them tend to promote their personal religious beliefs through their supposed ability to understand dreams. On the other hand, soulish interpretive methods, even those with some underlying spiritual basis, tend to be clothed in much more culturally neutral trappings, such as the science of psychology.

The primary proponents of soulish dream interpretation over the latter half of the twentieth century were Freud, Jung, and Perls (the founder of gestalt therapy). Of these three, Freud is perhaps the most recognizable, but Jung may have had the most impact on the Christian community's reluctance to accept biblical dream interpretation as a valid spiritual gift. This is because Jung's ungodly methods of interpreting dreams somehow managed to invade the Church and become socially acceptable for a season before their negative impact was fully recognized. Freud focused on psychoanalysis, Jung on archetypes, and Perls on projections, but none sought the true underlying *spiritual* significance of dreams, and thus their techniques were rooted in the soul's attempt to understand spiritual things. Being in complete contention with the Scriptures, such methods are destined for failure:

> *The natural person does not accept the things of the Spirit of God, for they are folly to him, and he is not able to understand them because they are spiritually discerned.* —1 Corinthians 2:14 (ESV)

It is only by his reliance upon the Holy Spirit's wisdom that man can ever hope to understand dreams at all. For this reason, because dependence on the Holy Spirit is essential, forms and formulas—whether couched in spiritual terminology or secular—will eventually fail. God will never allow us to become self-sufficient in the realm of dream interpretation (nor, for that matter, in any other area), but He will always draw us back to an understanding of our dependence upon Him. Without His guidance and revelation, we cannot interpret dreams (John 15:5), but with Him, not only does the interpretation of dreams become possible (Philippians 4:13), it becomes a source of life, strength, and hope.

Dream Stories by Michael B. French

Dreams of
Famous and Historical People

Not only have dreams played a significant role in the Scriptures, but they have also had a significant impact upon life throughout history. Having established the value of dreams and visions in the New Testament, it is helpful to recognize that their presence in the lives of believers has continued to impact the Church from the first century to the present day. Dreams have played an important role in the life and growth of the Church, but they have also had significant impact upon the culture around us. The biblical evidence for the value of dreams stands alone, but it is helpful to see how the understanding of their significance has been maintained over the years. Considering the value placed upon dreams by those closest to the New Testament era, it is difficult to imagine how this significance was ever lost.

To help us better understand how dreams have continued to have an impact upon the lives of those who follow Christ, it would be helpful to review some of the historical evidence in their favor. Each of the following anecdotes concerning dreams recounted by historical figures adds to the volume of evidence that dreams have significant value; however, each of them is also related in some fashion to a religious understanding of dreams. In order to more fully establish the overall value of dreams, it seems that some review of their cultural relevance would also be beneficial. Also included are anecdotes from more modern people whose dreams inspired creativity and invention in a very real and relevant cultural way.

Polycarp (69–155 AD): Polycarp, the bishop of the church of Smyrna, is one of the earliest and best known of all the followers of Jesus not named in the New Testament. He was one of the apostle John's disciples, and the account of his martyrdom is presented in *The Martyrdom of Polycarp.* According to the accounts making up this letter, three days before his arrest, Polycarp had a dream in which his pillow was in flames. He awoke and told those gathered with him that "I will be burnt alive"—accurately prophesying both his martyrdom and its means as a result of the dream. On the strength of this dream, Polycarp welcomed those who came to arrest him and offered them food and drink. He asked them to give him an hour of uninterrupted prayer, and then he would go with them. They gave him two hours, questioning why they had been put to the trouble of arresting such a godly old man. Instead of begging for his life, Polycarp was begged by the proconsul to denounce Christ so that he could set the old man free, to which Polycarp famously replied, "Eighty-six years have I served Him and He has done me no wrong. How can I blaspheme my King and my Savior?" Polycarp was then threatened with death by the release of wild animals, and when that did not seem to impact him, he was told he would be burned alive. Undoubtedly remembering his dream, he declared, "You threaten me with fire, which burns for an hour and is then extinguished, but you know nothing of the fire of the coming judgment and eternal punishment, reserved for the ungodly. Why are you waiting? Bring on whatever you want."[2]

Tertullian (160–225 AD): Tertullian, the son of a Roman centurion, was born in North Africa. He probably practiced law for a season before being converted to Christianity and apparently becoming a priest. It is among Tertullian's writings that the Latin word for *trinity* was first used to describe one God in three persons. Though accused of heresy late in his life, he and his writings are still considered a powerful witness to the faith. This early Church father was among the first to write extensively on the subject of spiritual dreams. In his *Treatise on the Soul*, Tertullian dealt with this subject throughout chapters 44 through 49. Tertullian took the position that not receiving dreams from God was actually a judgment upon the unbeliever. By implication, it would appear that he simply assumed that believers would naturally have dreams. Furthermore, Tertullian wrote, "It would not be unreasonable for a man to receive admonition from the Divine Being either in the way of warning or of alarm, as by a flash of lightning, or by a sudden stroke of death; only it would be [a] much more natural conclusion to believe that this process should be by a dream." It was also this Church father who might have been the first to espouse the sources of dreams as originating from three categories: 1) those inspired by demons, 2) those poured out by God, and 3) those the soul apparently creates for itself. From Tertullian's perspective, "almost the greater part of mankind get[s] their knowledge of God from dreams."[3]

Constantine (272–337 AD): Constantine was the first Roman emperor to support Christianity. Under his rule, Christianity was accepted as a Roman religion. There are mixed views on the impact that Constantine had on Christianity, with some feeling that it opened the doors of the faith and others feeling that its widespread political acceptance was detrimental. Regardless of how his impact on Christianity is seen, it was Constantine who formally ended the persecution of Christians and granted religious freedom through the issuance of the Edict of Milan in AD 313. Given his political and cultural position, Constantine's decision, that Christianity was to become his personal faith, is of monumental historical significance. In the spring of 312 AD, while campaigning against his rival, Maxentius, Constantine had a dream that convinced him of this decision.[4] The writings of Constantine's contemporaries differ on what the dream contained, but the most common accounts state that he saw a cross of light and was told to go and conquer by this sign. He went on to defeat Maxentius's superior force and attributed that victory to the God of Christianity, who had given him the dream the night before.

Synesius of Cyrene (370–413 AD): Synesius of Cyrene was a highly educated Greek intellectual who became the bishop of Ptolemais. He wrote *De Insomniis* (or, *On Dreams*), which continues to be influential in the Greek Orthodox Church today. In this writing, Synesius defended the idea that man had the capacity to foretell the future through the dreams he received. In addition, he identified very specific functions of dreams that he himself had experienced. "Often have they [dreams] aided me to put my ideas in order, and my style in harmony with my ideas. . . . At other times, in the hunting season, I invented, after a dream, traps to catch the swiftest animals and the most skillful in hiding . . . dreams would give me courage . . ."[5]

Saint Thomas Aquinas (1225–1274 AD): Saint Thomas Aquinas was an Italian Dominican friar, philosopher, and theologian. He was a prolific writer, penning more than sixty known works. Although Aquinas might have unwittingly helped to advance the concepts that led to the devaluing of dreams in his examination and discussion of

Aristotle's writings, he clearly believed that dreams were a valid means of revelation when received from God. His most profound and well-known work is called *Summa Theologica*. His conclusion on dreams was that:

> *We must say that there is no unlawful divination in making use of dreams for the foreknowledge of the future, so long as those dreams are due to divine revelation, or to some natural cause inward or outward, and so far as the efficacy of that cause extends. But it will be an unlawful and superstitious divination if it be caused by a revelation of the demons, with whom a compact has been made, whether explicit, through their being invoked for the purpose, or implicit, through the divination extending beyond its possible limits.[6]*

The position that Aquinas took indicated that dreams sometimes come from within and sometimes they come from without. Regarding dreams that originate from within, he saw them as either coming from the soul or the body. Regarding dreams that originate from without, he saw them as either being affected by the dreamer's surroundings or by spiritual things (either coming from God or from the demonic realm).[7] Despite its twenty-one volumes, *Summa Theologica* remains an unfinished work. On December 6, 1273, after experiencing an unusually long "ecstasy" (a term used to connote "dream" or "vision"), Thomas Aquinas laid his pen aside and wrote no more. When urged to continue his writings, he replied, "I can do no more. Such secrets have been revealed to me that all I have written now appears to be of little value."[8]

Paul McCartney: One of the most popular songs ever written by one of the most popular bands that ever wrote music is "Yesterday," performed by the Beatles. The legend of the song holds that Paul McCartney composed the entire melody from a dream he had one evening in 1964. *The Beatles Anthology* includes the following description in its notes, written by McCartney regarding the process of composing this song:

> *I was living in a little flat at the top of a house and I had a piano by my bed. I woke up one morning with a tune in my head and I thought, "Hey, I don't know this tune—or do I?" It was like a jazz melody. . . . I went to the piano and found the chords to it, made sure I remembered it, and then hawked it 'round to all my friends, asking what it was: "Do you know this? It's a good little tune, but I couldn't have written it, because I dreamt it."*

McCartney worried initially that he had subconsciously plagiarized someone else's work, but he eventually decided that, because no one else had claimed it, he could use it.[9]

Christopher Nolan: For the inspiration of the 2010 motion picture *Inception*, director Christopher Nolan seems to have looked to the lucid dreams of his childhood. In an interview with the *Los Angeles Times*, Nolan confessed that *Inception* was an elusive dream that he had wanted to turn into a movie since around the age of sixteen. According to the article, "Ever since he was a youngster, he says, he was intrigued by the way he would wake up and then, while he fell back into a lighter sleep, hold on to the awareness that he was, in fact, dreaming. Then there was the even more fascinating feeling that he could study the place and tilt the events of the dream."[10]

Edgar Allan Poe: The poet and writer Edgar Allan Poe is said to have been inspired to write several short stories from dreams that he had, and he actually wrote several poems about dreams, including "Dream-Land" and "A Dream Within a Dream." In 1839, he composed an essay entitled "An Opinion on Dreams," in which he described dreams as a powerful form of consciousness. He was a strong supporter of the divine nature of dreams, writing that "dreams, or, as they were then generally called, *visions*, were a means of supernatural instruction, if we believe the Bible at all, is proved by Jacob's dream, the several visions of Ezekiel and other prophets, as also of later date, the Revelations to Saint John; and there appears no reason why this mode of divine communication should be discontinued in the present day."[11]

Otto Loewi: While the name Otto Loewi might not be as familiar to most people as the names Nolan, Poe, or McCartney, without the work of Loewi, the advancements we have seen in modern neurology would have be severely hindered. Loewi was born in Germany in 1873, and he became a professor of pharmacology at the University of Graz in the Austrian Alps in 1909. In 1921, he conducted a groundbreaking experiment that eventually won him a share of the 1936 Nobel Prize in Medicine. (It was also awarded to his friend Henry Dale.) The prize was awarded for demonstrating chemical neurotransmission, which many consider to be the origin of neurology itself.

The story of how Loewi devised the now-classical experiment is that of a dream. In the wee hours of the morning on Easter Sunday 1920, Loewi awoke from a dream and scribbled a few notes on a scrap of paper. The next morning when he arose, he was horrified to discover that he could not read his own handwriting. He spent the remainder of the day desperately, but unsuccessfully, trying to reconstruct his dream. When he was finally able to fall asleep again that night, he once again dreamed of the experiment, awoke from his dream, and in much more careful handwriting, wrote out the steps he had dreamt. He then arose and went immediately to his laboratory to conduct the experiment he had just completed in his dream, and the results of the experiment proved the chemical nature of neurotransmission.[12]

Abraham Lincoln: The sixteenth president of the United States of America, Abraham Lincoln, was fatally shot by John Wilkes Booth on April 14, 1865, while attending a play at Ford's Theater in Washington, D.C. On April 11th, he told his close friend Ward Hill Lamon that he had experienced a dream that had "strangely annoyed" him since he'd had it a week prior. Lincoln recounted his dream as follows:[13]

> *About ten days ago, I retired very late. I had been up waiting for important dispatches from the front. I could not have been long in bed when I fell into a slumber, for I was weary. I soon began to dream. There seemed to be a deathlike stillness about me. Then I heard subdued sobs, as if a number of people were weeping. I thought I left my bed and wandered downstairs. There the silence was broken by the same pitiful sobbing, but the mourners were invisible. I went from room to room; no living person was in sight, but the same mournful sounds of distress met me as I passed along. I saw light in all the rooms; every object was familiar to me; but where were all the people who were grieving as if their hearts would break? I was puzzled and*

alarmed. What could be the meaning of all this? Determined to find the cause of a state of things so mysterious and so shocking, I kept on until I arrived at the East Room, which I entered. There I met with a sickening surprise. Before me was a catafalque, on which rested a corpse wrapped in funeral vestments. Around it were stationed soldiers who were acting as guards; and there was a throng of people, gazing mournfully upon the corpse, whose face was covered, others weeping pitifully. "Who is dead in the White House?" I demanded of one of the soldier. "The president," was his answer. "He was killed by an assassin." Then came a loud burst of grief from the crowd, which woke me from my dream. I slept no more that night; and although it was only a dream, I have been strangely annoyed by it ever since.

It is also said that Lamon, Lincoln's friend and law partner, described Byron's "The Dream" as one of Lincoln's favorite poems, and he indicated that the president would often repeat the following lines:

Sleep hath its own world,
A boundary between the things misnamed
Death and existence: Sleep hath its own world,
And a wide realm of wild reality,
And dreams in their development have breath,
And tears, and tortures, and the touch of joy;
They leave a weight upon our waking thoughts,
They take a weight from off waking toils,
They do divide our being. [14]

Elias Howe: With the invention of the sewing machine, everyday life was radically changed. While a number of people had worked on the idea over many years, Elias Howe is ultimately considered the inventor of this life-changing, everyday piece of machinery. Born in Massachusetts in 1819, Howe was wise enough to put together all of the ideas of those who had worked on this project before him with his own innovations *and* a design for the needle that he had received in a dream. Between 1856 and 1867, when his patent expired, Howe earned at least $2,000,000 in license fees. Prior to Howe's sewing machine, the primary method of sewing involved a handheld needle pulled through the cloth with the eye of the needle as the last part to go through. This, however, was not working for the sewing machine designs. Howe went to bed late one night after an extended effort to resolve the problem of the thread not catching correctly. That night he dreamed of natives in a jungle who threw him into a stewpot. While he tried to escape in the dream, he noticed that all the natives had spears with which they were poking him. Later that day after awakening, as he pondered the dream, he realized that all of the natives' spears had holes in their tips—and thus the problem of the sewing machine needle was resolved.[15]

Madam C.J. Walker: Born in 1867 to former slaves, Sarah Breedlove would be named the first self-made American female millionaire by the *Guinness Book of World Records.* However, this distinction came after she married newspaperman Charles Joseph Walker and changed her name to Madam C.J. Walker. She considered this new name to have a sophisticated sound that would instill confidence in shoppers. The means of her success would be Madam Walker's Wonderful Hair Grower scalp conditioner. At the age of seven, she had been orphaned, and by the age of nineteen, she was supporting herself and her daughter as a washerwoman. In her early thirties, she found that her hair was falling out, and she desperately sought a way to make it regrow. No hair products on the market worked, so she decided to create one herself. She had no success, until one day, as she told a reporter, "God answered my prayer, for one night I had a dream, and in that dream a big black man appeared to me and told me what to mix up for my hair. Some of the remedy was grown in Africa, but I sent for it, mixed it up, put it on my scalp, and in a few weeks my hair was coming in faster than it had ever fallen out. I tried it on my friends; it helped them. I made up my mind I would begin to sell it."[16]

Samuel Taylor Coleridge: Samuel Taylor Coleridge indicated that one of his most famous poems came to him in a dream. He even titled it "Kubla Khan: Or a Vision in a Dream." By his own account, he was ill and had taken a medicine, an opiate, to help him sleep. Whatever the cause, Coleridge claimed to have entered a profound sleep and dreamt hundreds of lines of the poem. Unfortunately, upon awakening and beginning to write, he was interrupted by a visitor, and when he returned to complete the poem, he could remember it no more. The poet's account is found in the preface to the poem:

> *In the summer of the year 1797, the Author, then in ill health, had retired to a lonely farmhouse between Porlock and Linton, on the Exmoor confines of Somerset and Devonshire. In consequence of a slight indisposition, an anodyne had been prescribed, from the effects of which he fell asleep in his chair at the moment that he was reading the following sentence, or words of the same substance, in "Purchas's Pilgrimage:" "Here the Khan Kubla commanded*

a palace to be built, and a stately garden thereunto. And thus ten miles of fertile ground were inclosed [sic] with a wall." The author continued for about three hours in a profound sleep, at least of the external senses, during which time he had the most vivid confidence, that he could not have composed less than from two to three hundred lines; if that indeed can be called composition in which all the images rose up before him as things, with a parallel production of the correspondent expressions, without any sensation or consciousness of effort. On awaking he appeared to himself to have a distinct recollection of the whole, and taking his pen, ink, and paper, instantly and eagerly wrote down the lines that are here preserved. At this moment he was unfortunately called out by a person on business from Porlock, and detained by him above an hour, and on his return to his room, found to his no small surprise and mortification, that though he still retained some vague and dim recollection of the general purpose of the vision, yet, with the exception of some eight or ten scattered lines and images, all the rest had passed away like the images on the surface of a stream into which a stone has been cast. . . .[17]

Some people have described dreams as being "written in disappearing ink," and it would appear that this description is quite valid. One of the great lessons learned from Coleridge's experience can be found in the need to record a dream as quickly as possible after its experience.

Jasper Johns: The work of artist Jasper Johns has impacted the art world since the 1950s. Born in Augusta, Georgia, in 1930, Johns broke out of the world of abstract expressionism in 1954 by painting a recognizable everyday object, the American flag. Drawing from the brushstroke style of the abstract expressionists, his work blurred the lines between fine art and everyday life. Johns recounts that the image came to him in a dream: "One night I dreamed I painted a large American flag, and the next morning I got up and I went out and bought the materials to begin it. And I did. I worked on that painting for a long time. It's a very rotten painting—physically rotten—because I began it in house enamel paint, which you paint furniture with, and it wouldn't dry quickly enough. Then I had in my head this idea of something I had read or heard about: wax encaustic." The painting launched Johns to the forefront of the art world.[18]

Jack Nicklaus: As of 2015, Jack Nicklaus had remained third on the list of the all-time greatest winners in the world of golf. This distinction did not take into consideration the fact that Nicklaus had only played a limited schedule of tour events each year, choosing to focus largely on the major tournaments. Known as the "Golden Bear," Nicklaus is considered to be one of the greatest professional golfers to have ever played the game. However, even the greatest among us in any endeavor go through challenging or difficult times, and Nicklaus was no exception. After posting a series of bad scores in tournaments during the 1964 season, he rallied and turned things around. Explaining the change in a newspaper interview, Nicklaus said: "Wednesday night I had a dream, and it was about my golf swing. I was hitting them pretty good in the dream, and all at once I realized I wasn't holding the club the way

I've actually been holding it lately. I've been having trouble collapsing my right arm, taking the club head away from the ball, but I was doing it perfectly in my sleep. So, when I came to the course yesterday morning, I tried it the way I did in my dream and it worked. I shot a 68 yesterday and a 65 today."[19]

The Voice, Season 10 (2016): NBC's hit show *The Voice* entered its tenth season with an interesting twist on how dreams impact everyday life. On the second night of the blind auditions segment, a young singer by the name of Lacy Mandigo entered the competition singing the song "Son of a Preacher Man," originally recorded by Dusty Springfield in 1968.

As Lacy began to sing the last note, none of the musical celebrities had selected her for their team, but at the last possible moment, Christina Aguilera selected Lacy for her team. After Lacy's initial excitement, she declared with joy, "I had a dream last night that you turned around for me, and it was on the very last note," to which Aguilera responded, "And now it happened."[20] As if that was not enough, when the time came for her to go head-to-head with her fellow contestant Allison Porter, Lacy was released from Aguilera's team in tears, only to hear the buzzer sound as she was "stolen" by Blake Shelton, thus allowing her to continue in the competition. Through her tears, she told Aguilera, "Remember that time I told you that I dreamed you were the only one that turned around? I dreamed the other night that Blake saved me. I swear to God."[21] As if in recognition of the power of dreams, both Adam Levine and Pharrell Williams began to ask if she could dream that she would ultimately end up on their teams, as well.

Others: Salvador Dali frequently described his paintings as "hand-painted dream photographs." John Lennon's song

"#9 Dream" repeats a nonsense phrase from a dream in its chorus and contains the lyrics to describe it: "So long ago/Was it in a dream, was it just a dream?/Seemed so very real, it seemed so real to me." Handel is said to have composed his classic *Messiah* from the chorus he first discerned in a dream, and Albert Einstein's groundbreaking theory of relativity has been mythically attributed to a dream.

Interpreting Dreams

With the significance of dreams established, the issue of how can they be interpreted becomes a topic of some importance. As was addressed briefly in the first chapter, the psychology and New Age avenues of interpretation seem of little value in identifying the life-giving meanings of dreams, especially those that are inspired by Holy Spirit. Just as we can identify three sources for dreams, it would seem that those same three sources could be used for the interpretation of dreams: God, our own souls, and our adversary. The psychological methods of dream interpretation arise from our own souls' attempts to understand the mysteries of a dream without the assistance of Holy Spirit. The New Age and eastern religion–inspired attempts draw upon the spiritual realm, but unfortunately, they pull from the demonic realm rather than the godly one. Neither of these methods can give life to the message of a dream. Without the Spirit of God getting involved, a dream's interpretation will always fall flat to one degree or another, whether in its impact or in its reception.

The first rule of Spirit-led dream interpretation is that there are no rules. If we are seeking a formula that, when applied, will always lead to a correct spiritual interpretation, then we are pursuing a method that has not been established by God. Consider the nature of mankind—if a foolproof method of systematic dream interpretation were to exist, it would immediately eliminate our need to depend on the Holy Spirit. As soon as I become certain that a particular symbol can always be interpreted to mean a particular thing, God will use it in a new and unique way in order to ensure my continued need to seek understanding from His Spirit. Certain biblical principles of interpretation do exist, but they can never take the form of fixed rules when it comes to actual interpretation, though they may be absolute when it comes to God's nature. For example, it is absolutely fixed that any dream interpretation that attempts to steer the dreamer away from the established principles of God's Word is not a valid interpretation. This is a fixed principle of interpretation, rather than a rule that governs how to interpret a specific dream.

Many resources exist that offer assistance in understanding dreams, including various forms of dream symbol dictionaries. It is important to understand that while these can be valuable resources, they do not establish unerring formulas. As long as human beings are involved in the interpretive process, there is always the possibility of error and even the misapplication of principle. We can consider the idea of dream dictionaries as an illustration of this point. A myriad of resources exists purporting to identify the common symbols found in dreams and provide a short list of their common meanings. Such resources, in and of themselves, are not a problem, and they can provide helpful insight into the world of dream interpretation; however, when they are used as a dictionary to interpret every dream a person has, they can become problematic. The term *dictionary* implies that we should be able to look up a particular symbol and its specific meaning or meanings for every instance that symbol appears. The assumption would be that one or more of these meanings could then be applied as the correct meaning of that symbol each and every time. The temptation is to then apply that definition of a symbol just as we would apply the definition of a word, and thereby grasp the meaning of the dream as we would come to the understanding of the meaning of a sentence. In many cases, this may work well; yet, if taken to an extreme, it can ultimately eliminate our dependence on the Holy Spirit in favor of the dream dictionary. It is almost certain that when a person becomes dependent on human resources instead of on the Holy Spirit, the Father God will take some type of step to remove that dependence.

A symbol in any particular dream may have a meaning so personal in nature that we need the Holy Spirit to reveal its onetime, personal meaning for a particular dreamer, or we risk misunderstanding the entire dream. We can also run into the issue of metaphors, which are vital to the understanding of a dream, but which are nowhere to be found in any human resource or list of potential meanings. This was precisely the case when a chance encounter at a public festival led to the interpretation of an interesting dream. The dreamer was a young man who looked like a high school or college football linebacker and who displayed that "macho jock" personality that one might expect. He was surrounded by a group of young people who appeared to be his teammates and cheerleaders, when the following opportunity for dream interpretation occurred.

"I dreamed I was being slapped in the face with biscuits," declared the young man. Yes, this was the entire dream. We can learn many techniques to help take the time we need to hear the Holy Spirit when we are preparing to share an interpretation; however, none of them seemed to work in this case. Asking the dreamer for further clarification or to repeat the dream provided substantially no additional time for the interpreter to listen for God's voice. Recalling multiple dream lists and interpretive resources provided no support, either, as there seemed to be no recollection of "biscuits" being listed in any of them. These was an instance when all formulas failed and the dream dictionaries came up lacking. Such a time requires those who interpret dreams to be quick to hear the Holy Spirit give His understanding. In a desperate move to gain another few moments to listen for the Spirit's voice, the interpreter asked, "Were they canned or homemade biscuits?" to which the dreamer, without hesitation, responded, "Homemade!" In an instant, without any support from a man-made dictionary definition, the meaning became clear, and the interpreter informed the dreamer that there were issues that were causing him conflict with his mother. He needed to go to her and resolve the situation. The response was priceless, as this large, macho jock broke down in tears, right in front of his peers, acknowledging that the interpretation of the dream had pierced his heart.

No dictionary or formula could ever have achieved this result. It was powerful, but the symbols were very personal and unique to this particular dream and to the dreamer. The Holy Spirit was the only Source that could have provided such an interpretation as this.

Symbols may have specific biblical meanings, cultural meanings, colloquial meanings, or even personal meanings that cannot be relegated to an overarching formula, definition, or list of meanings. With such varied possibilities from which to draw meaning, even having such amazing resources at our fingertips as we do requires that we remain dependent on Holy Spirit for when to use them and for which ones to use. Lists, books, teachings, and our own experiences can be drawn upon as the Holy Spirit calls them to our recollection. After all, the Holy Spirit is not only the One who teaches us how to interpret dreams; He is the One who reminds us of the pieces we need to assemble in order to interpret dreams successfully (see John 14:26). It may be helpful to think of the resources that are available to assist us with interpretation as files in a computer database. When we are confronted with a particular symbol in a dream, such as a kitchen table, we can open the folder labeled *Dream Symbols*, then navigate through the various subfolders, *Furniture > Kitchen Furniture > Tables*, until we find a list of possible meanings. We can then ask the Holy Spirit which meaning applies, but we also need to be prepared for Him to say, "None of them."

Understanding the symbols of a dream as we seek an interpretation also involves recognizing the process of how each symbol relates to the other elements of the dream, as well. In the world of real estate, it is said that the value of a piece of property is determined by three things: *location, location, location.* In the world of dream interpretation, the meaning of a particular symbol is significantly impacted by three things: *context, context, context.* For example, whether the understanding of a symbol should be considered positive or negative will often be determined by the context in which the symbol is found, rather than by the presence of the metaphor itself.

It can become very easy to assume that we know what a particular symbol should mean, but the context of the dream itself can often help us to see the metaphor in a different light. Consider the following symbols and their most probable, natural meanings:

> A large, ominous-looking blackbird
> A small, brilliantly colored bluebird

Before reading further, stop for a moment and reach a determination in your own mind as to what you think the most likely meaning of these two symbols would be.

Selah: pause and think before continuing.

In most cases, any individual asked this question will bring some level of preconception to the decision-making process. Such preconceptions would typically be influenced by natural perceptions of color and size. Thus, it is more likely that the blackbird would be viewed in a negative light and the bluebird in a more positive one. If you were aware that birds can often represent spiritual beings, then it might be quite normal to assume that the blackbird would be a demonic influence and the bluebird would be more of a godly symbol. But now stop and consider the same symbols in the context of a hypothetical dream:

> *In my dream, I was sitting in my room, and there was a small bird perched on my shoulder. It was a beautiful bird, brilliant blue in color. As I sat listening to its song, I seemed to grow weary, as though a tremendous weight had settled over me. Just when I thought I could take no more, a large and rather ominous-looking blackbird flew into the room. When it did, the little bluebird jumped from my shoulder and flew out the window. The large blackbird dropped something on the table in front of me, and I knew that it wanted me to eat it. I picked up what appeared to be a crumb of bread, and when I ate it, the weariness seemed to leave me and I began to feel much better.*

If you are like most people, even as you read this hypothetical dream, your perception of the meaning of the two symbols began to quickly shift. Inherently, it now seems that the bluebird might have been more of a negative symbol and the blackbird more of a positive one. Suddenly, the context allows us to see the blackbird more in relationship to the story of the ravens that fed Elijah (see 1 Kings 17:4–6). While blue can be a beautiful color, it is also frequently associated with depression, and here, the context of the dream nudges us in a direction to see this small bluebird more in the light of that understanding.

Dreams need interpretation in order to have value, and a dream cannot be interpreted properly without a dependence on the Holy Spirit for the inspiration. While men may interpret the dream, it is God who gives the interpretation. This is exactly the point Joseph was making when he asked the cupbearer, "Do not interpretations belong to God?" (Genesis 40:8 NIV). Daniel described things in much the same light when he told King Nebuchadnezzar that the "wisdom of men was insufficient for the interpretation of dreams..." (Daniel 2:28 NIV).

These examples of how an interpretation is dependent upon the leading of the Holy Spirit provide the primary illustration of the difference between a Spirit interpretation and a soulish or a demonic one. While there are certainly other distinctions that can be made, the way an interpreter approaches the understanding of the dream symbols sets the tone for which source the interpretation will be drawn from. A spiritual interpretation to any dream, whether it be from God, from the soul, or from the enemy, will produce life. On the other hand, even if the dream is from God, a soulish or demonically inspired interpretation will drain the life out of it. By keeping these concepts in mind, the dream stories contained in the second part of this book will provide benefit beyond merely interesting reading, and they will become useful as valuable lessons on dream interpretation.

Categories of Dreams

While there are only a limited number of possible sources for dreams, the general nature of the messages contained by dreams could be categorized any number of ways. In an effort to help bring order to this far-reaching topic, the twenty categories of dreams, as first identified by John Paul Jackson in his course entitled *Understanding Dreams and Visions*[22] and which are now the topic of a book entitled *The 20 Categories of Dreams: Understanding the Various Ways God Speaks Through Dreams* by Michael Wise[23], will be used to help drive our discussion.

The categories discussed below are by no means exhaustive, and you may feel more comfortable with other or additional descriptions. They do, however, provide a starting place for discussion. It can be argued that there are too many categories listed, just as easily as it can be argued there are too few. Use these categories for the purpose for which they are intended: to provide a starting point for discussion and examination of individual dreams. In this way, they can help us to better identify the source of a dream and to come to a foundational understanding of what the dream may be about and how to respond to it.

It should also be pointed out that dreams do not fit nicely into individual categories. It is likely that any given dream could be put into multiple categories and/or that different individuals could place any given dream into a different category than what has been chosen for this book. Do not allow these differences to impact the use of these resources. Recognize that the categories described below and used for the real-life dream stories included herein are simply a starting point for your journey and not a finish line for how you should think.

In most cases, the category names themselves will provide a basic idea of what the dreams in that category are related to, however, a brief description is also provided in order to help provide more specific understanding of the type of dreams that would be included in each category.

Healing Dreams: These are dreams that provide some form of healing. This may include physical, mental, relational, emotional, spiritual, or other types of healing. Healing may be received in the dream itself and manifest upon the person awakening, or the dream can be the signal that healing has begun and it should continue upon waking. Unless God is the Source of the dream, however, it will not be a true healing dream.

Self-Condition Dreams: These are dreams that help us to understand something about ourselves. They often include some element(s) that help us to see where we are as opposed to where God wants us to be. When these dreams are from God, they provide hope for reaching the "condition" in which God wants us to be.

Calling Dreams: These are dreams that help us to recognize the call of God on our lives. They may identify either a general or a specific vocation or ministry that we are to pursue. These dreams can also help us to recognize and begin to pursue our true destiny. When they come from God, these dreams usually provide hope that we can become the person God created us to be.

Courage Dreams: These are dreams designed to strengthen us in our faith or encourage us that we are capable of accomplishing something that God has given us to do. Courage dreams are edifying in nature, and they help us to believe in ourselves and in the God who enables and empowers us to overcome the challenges we face. These dreams are rarely from the enemy (and never in a believer's life), because they propel dreamers forward in God's plans for their lives.

Direction Dreams: These are dreams that give direction to the dreamer regarding a place to go (such as Joseph's dream to take the holy family to Egypt), a time to do something (such as Joseph's dream concerning when to return the holy family to Israel), or a change of plans (such as the Magis' dream to go home a different way from the way they had come to visit the newborn Savior). Even when these dreams are from God, it is often helpful to have additional confirmation before acting on the direction that is provided in the dream.

Intercessory Dreams: These are dreams that provide a call to prayer and give us instructions on how to pray. The need for prayer can be immediate, something that is needed in the near future, or even for needs that are distant in time or geography. Dreams that call us to prayer are never from the enemy and almost never originate from our own souls.

Invention Dreams: These are dreams that spark creativity. Dreams in this category can provide ideas for literal inventions or conceptual ideas, such as music, art, and dance. The function and use of the idea given in the dream can be either abused or redeemed, but such dreams can come from all three sources. Please note that the demonic world does not truly operate out of creativity, but rather by counterfeiting the creativity of the Lord.

Word of Knowledge Dreams: These are dreams that provide specific information, such as a solution to a problem or the answer to a question. Practically speaking, they are much like the spiritual gift identified as the word of knowledge, except the "word" is delivered through a dream. While the category name implies a spiritual gift, and thus we could assume that such dreams would always come from God, it should be noted that information (as opposed to revelation) can be conveyed through dreams by the enemy.

Prophetic Dreams: These are dreams that reveal the future. Practically speaking, these are prophetic words released in the form of a dream. Revelatory dreams are from God, as only He knows the future. The enemy may attempt to counterfeit this category of dreams, in the same way he would counterfeit the word of knowledge dreams, by making predictions based upon the limited information that he has.

Warning Dreams: These are dreams, as the name implies, that warn the dreamer not to take a certain action, or they provide insight into the dangers of a given situation. Dreams in this category tend to come from God.

Correction Dreams: These are dreams that provide the dreamer with insight into changing a given attitude, opinion, or behavior. When they come from God, they help dreamers to make course corrections in their lives. These dreams can help the dreamer recognize bad habits and patterns of corruption to which they are adhering. To distinguish the source of dreams in this category, remember that correction from God brings conviction, while harassment from the enemy is designed to bring condemnation.

Flushing Dreams: These are dreams that help dreamers let go of the little things they encounter throughout the day that would otherwise have a negative impact upon their lives. Brushes with the demonic that went almost unnoticed can be rejected and overcome through experiencing this type of dream. These are dreams from an omniscient God, who recognizes the issues that will impact our life, even if we do not.

Deliverance Dreams: These are dreams that release dreamers from more direct and recognizable demonic assaults in their lives. Just like deliverance in "real life" while the dreamer is awake, these dreams can both remove demonic attachments and provide relief from demonic oppression. These are dreams from God, who is directly intervening in the life of the dreamer to bring about greater freedom.

Spiritual Warfare Dreams: These are dreams that involve some sort of attack or warfare against the dreamer or others. They typically involve some level of fear, and they are often set in some form of life-or-death situation. These are dreams inspired by the demonic realm, in which the dreamer is often, if not always, losing the battle.

Fear Dreams: These are dreams that cause fear to arise in the life of the dreamer. Nightmares or night terrors are in this category of dreams. These are dreams inspired by the demonic realm, and they can either cause fear or be the result of living in fear, which opens a door to their assault.

False Dreams: These are dreams that oppose the plan of God in the dreamer's life. They often present the enemy's plans in an effort to cause the dreamer to see the fulfillment of the dream as inevitable. This category also includes a lie that recounts a dream that was never actually experienced, for the purpose of manipulation. These are dreams that are inspired by the demonic realm, and they are often birthed out of the soul. It is important for the dreamer to reject the lies presented in this category of dreams.

Dark Dreams: These are almost always black-and-white or gray-scale dreams, devoid of color. Such dreams are often intended to cause depression, destruction, or anxiety, as they reveal what the enemy intends to do in the dreamer's life. These dreams are inspired by the demonic realm, and they are an expression of the enemy's purpose: to kill, steal and destroy (see John 10:10).

Chemical Dreams: These are dreams that result from the chemical influence of drugs, alcohol, herbs, or various types of food. The proverbial "pizza dream" (as in, "I ate spicy food before going to bed and then had a strange dream") falls into this category. These are dreams that arise from the dreamer's soul, although the intake of the chemical causes of the dream may in some cases be at the provocation of the demonic realm.

Body Dreams: These are dreams that result from physical sickness or conditions of the body. High fever, pregnancy, and other medical conditions can provoke these disjointed and often confusing dreams. These dreams arise from the dreamer's soul, and they can be among the most difficult in which to find meaning.

Soul Dreams: These are dreams that result from our own personal feelings, thoughts, and desires. They are an outgrowth of the things for which our souls are longing. Oftentimes they result from what our souls are contending against our spirits for. These dreams arise from the dreamer's soul and are triggered by the intensity of the passion that inspires them.

PART 2
REAL DREAM STORIES

This section of the book provides numerous examples of real dreams, their interpretations, the impact they had on the lives of the dreamers, and some short lessons on what can be learned from them. The first two dream examples are taken from the Bible and are placed into the format used for the subsequent contemporary dreams, so that you can get a feel for how to use the materials contained herein. The remaining dreams are contemporary dreams from real people around the world. These dreams are provided not only to help you understand more about dreams, but also to provide further evidence of the modern-day value of dreams and biblical dream interpretation.

As you read the dreams described on the following pages, keep in mind that they are each taken from the real-life experiences of people just like you and me. When we look to history, as was done in the section on *Dreams of Famous and Historical People*, it is easy to assume that the amazing dream stories recorded here could never happen to the average person. This is because we are looking back at people whose lives rose above average, often at least in part due to their ability to hear God through dreams and in other ways. We can look to the past and see the impact that the dreams had on their lives, but when we look at contemporary examples of dreams, it is often the case that insufficient time has passed for any people but those directly affected to understand the impact that each dream has had. These stories are intended to encourage each of us, to help us remember that we can truly hear from God and that what we hear can, in fact, change our lives. After all, we all have a tendency to think that we could never do the things that Jesus did, but He Himself told us that we could "do the things that He did and even greater things" (see John 14:12). May the stories on the following pages not only inspire you to believe that dreams can edify, encourage, and comfort you, but may they also encourage you to remember that you can grow to be more like Jesus every day.

As you read through the dreams in this part of the book, the following terms, as used to format the presentation of the dreams, will be useful to understand:

Dream Title: Each dreamer was asked, "If your dream was to be written as a short story, what would its title be?" The exceptions to this are the first few dreams listed, which have been taken from the Scriptures. A title has been added to each of these dreams for the sake of consistency. Later titles, as provided by the dreamers themselves, help to point attention to the elements and metaphors contained in the dream or the feelings conveyed by the dream that were of most significance to the dreamer.

QR Code: Some dreams may have a "QR code" that you can use to hear the dreamer provide more details about the dream and its significance. If you do not have access to a QR code reader, the Web site associated with the QR code is listed in the index of this book.

Dreamer: This provides relevant information about the dreamer, without relinquishing his or her identity. In this way, the anonymity of the dreamer is preserved, but be aware that each dream is a *real* dream from a *real* person who can be identified specifically.

Source: This line identifies the source from which the dream originated. Typically, the source of the dream will be one of the following: God (a dream inspired by the Holy Spirit), the soul (a dream originating from the dreamer's own mind, will, or emotions), or the enemy (a dream inspired by the demonic realm).

Color: This line identifies the level of color found in the dream. This information is helpful in determining whether or not the dream is from God. First John 1:5 declares that God is light and there is no darkness in Him at all. Because real color comes from light, then perfect light would produce perfect color. The enemy, being a counterfeiter, operates from a place of darkness, and thus the colors he can inspire would be noticeably less vivid. Thus, dreams in black and white, in gray scale, or in muted colors tend to be inspired by the demonic realm.

Dream Category: This information helps to place the dream into one of the twenty listed dream categories previously described. As has already been noted and will become apparent in reading the dreams included, these categories are not "absolutes," and many (if not most) of the dreams could be placed into different or multiple categories as easily as the one they have been associated with in this section.

Dream: This recounts the dream in the words of the dreamer. To the extent possible, other than editing for clarity, the dream has not been changed from the dreamer's original submission.

Dreamer's Understanding/Interpretation: This provides the dreamer's understanding of what the dream meant to them, and/or what someone told them that the dream meant. Sometimes it is recounted in the dreamer's own words.

Author's Spirit-Led Interpretation: This information identifies a short, simple Spirit-led interpretation of the dream as provided by the author. In most cases, this interpretation is made without reference to the dreamer's understanding of the dream, although the two frequently line up and help to provide clarity for why/how the dream made an impact on the dreamer's life.

In some cases, the author's Spirit-led interpretation was provided to the dreamer prior to the fulfillment of the dream, and then it was adapted for use in this book. In other cases, an interpretation was provided by the author and obviously written after the dream's fulfillment. In these cases, every effort was made to convey the same interpretation in the same language that would have been used prior to the outcome being made known. Wherever possible, the author has interpreted the dream prior to being made aware of the final impact/outcome of the dream. In all cases, it was the dreamer who ultimately recognized how the dream was applicable to his or her own life. Furthermore, it is important to point out that an accurate interpretation can come before *or after* the fulfillment of the dream; however, an interpretation before the dream's fulfillment strengthens the testimony of the dream.

Impact/Outcome: This line attempts to outline briefly how the dream made an impact on the dreamer's life. In almost every case, the impact described is given in the words of the dreamer and has only been edited for clarity. It should be noted that some of the outcomes may be viewed by the reader as significant, while others may seem insignificant. Please remember that these dreams were submitted for inclusion by the dreamers because they personally felt that the impact the dream had on them was highly significant in their own personal experience.

Primary Metaphor(s): This contains a selection of the most obvious or most significant metaphors from each dream and their meanings in the dream as submitted. The metaphors and meanings listed herein should not be used to compile a "dictionary" for the reasons previously addressed, but they can be used to help the reader gain a greater understanding of how symbols are used by the Holy Spirit and how their natural meanings can assist in dreamers in reaching an understanding of why the Holy Spirit used them.

Lesson: This will generally contain thoughts to help the reader understand basic principles of the biblical dream interpretation process. These will, by necessity, be limited in their scope, and in most cases, they will focus only on no more than two or three lessons from each dream, though many dreams may provide an opportunity to address far more concepts. For further information on the process of biblical dream interpretation, please refer to the resources listed in the *Authors' Acknowledgments* section at the end of this book.

***

The pages that follow include contemporary testimonies of how different dreams have changed people's lives. Before jumping directly into the stories of people just like us, however, two "example dreams" from the Scriptures are provided. These dreams provide an illustration of how the rest of the dreams in this section flow, and they provide further encouragement that the God of the dreams of the Bible is the same God who speaks in the same way (through dreams and visions) to His people today.

Visit
www.MyDreamStories.com

Example Dream: Pouring Wine Again

Dreamer: A male butler or cupbearer in Egypt

Source: God

Color: Unknown, but likely in color

Dream Category: Courage

Dream: In my dream, there was a vine before me, and on the vine, there were three branches. As soon as it budded, its blossoms shot forth and the clusters ripened into grapes. Pharaoh's cup was in my hand, and I took the grapes and pressed them into Pharaoh's cup and placed the cup in Pharaoh's hand. Taken from Genesis 40:9–11.

Dreamer's Understanding/Interpretation: Without an interpretation, this dream left the dreamer troubled and downcast (Genesis 40:6–7).

Author's Spirit-Led Interpretation: The three branches are three days. In three days, Pharaoh will lift up your head and restore you to your office, and you shall place Pharaoh's cup in his hand as you did formerly, when you were his cupbearer (Genesis 40:12–13).

Impact/Outcome: The dreamer took courage and was soon restored to his previous position (Genesis 40:21).

Primary Metaphor(s):

Three branches—three days

Budded—new life

Cup in hand—restoration

Lesson: Some dreams contain metaphors that are difficult to grasp unless either they are revealed totally by the Holy Spirit or the interpreter has some understanding of the cultural context in which the dream is received. It is important to keep in mind that God uses multiple methods of conveying the correct understanding of any given symbol. It is not necessary to hear an audible voice from heaven in order to describe the meaning of a particular metaphor, although that is, in fact, one method that God has and can use. The meaning of a symbol can become known in several ways, such as being revealed within the dream itself, by hearing the still, small voice of God, by seeing its meaning in the mind's eye, through the natural understanding of its use or purpose, through an understanding of colloquial usage, or through any number of other ways. In the cultural, geographical, and historical context of this dream, each cluster or branch of grapes would have provided approximately enough wine for Pharaoh for one day. Joseph would have most likely been familiar with this concept, if not from his experiences during his time in Egypt, then perhaps from his interactions with the wine bearer himself. By allowing God to draw his attention to something he quite possibly already knew, the meaning of the symbol was revealed.

Example Dream B: Bringing in the Sheaves

Dreamer: Joseph in Canaan

Source: God

Color: Unknown, buLt probably color

Dream Category: Calling dream

Dream: We were binding sheaves in the field, and behold, my sheaf arose and stood upright. And behold, your sheaves gathered around it and bowed down to my sheaf. Taken from Genesis 37:6–7.

Dreamer's Understanding/Interpretation: Joseph's brothers understood the dream to mean that Joseph felt he would rule over them (Genesis 37:8).

Author's Spirit-Led Interpretation: There is no direct scriptural interpretation of this dream, but the following interpretation is certainly implied: God was going to position Joseph in a place of authority over even those in his own family who currently had authority over him.

Impact/Outcome: Joseph was sold into slavery, but ultimately he was positioned in Egypt as a leader second only to Pharaoh. This position allowed him to save the lives of his family members and literally found his brothers bowing down to him.

Primary Metaphor(s):

Sheaves—provision, or in this case, Joseph's family members

Bowed down—honoring another

Lesson: One of the most significant lessons that can be gleaned from this dream is that not all dreams are for sharing; some are just for personal prayer. It is important to remember that while it would be impossible to discern an actual statistical number of the percentage of dreams that are more for prayer than to share, experience would indicate that if it was possible, the number would be very high, perhaps as much as 95 percent. One reason for this is the ease with which dreamers in our Western culture tend to fall into the trap of taking credit for something God is doing or of seeking recognition for themselves due to something that God has said.

In Joseph's case, it is likely that he already knew he was envied by his brothers in light of Genesis 37:4, which explains how they could not speak peaceably to him. Certainly, after seeing their reaction to this dream, Joseph should have become aware that he did not have the favor necessary to share his dreams before he communicated the second dream about the sun, moon, and stars found in verse 9. It quite possibly would have been more advantageous for Joseph to simply pray about his dreams and trust God to bring them to pass without sharing them with his family.

Certainly, we know that God used Joseph's sharing of this dream to ultimately position him in Egypt, but there were clearly other ways that God could have delivered him there that would have been much easier on Joseph. However, in the economy of God's Kingdom nothing is wasted, and all that resulted from this dream prepared

Joseph for the task that was set before him. It took many years for this dream to come to pass; it did not happen quickly, and as the psalmist wrote (see Psalm 105:19), during all the time it had not yet been fulfilled, the dream tested Joseph, and that testing brought about growth in his life.

Dream Stories by Michael B. French

Dream 1:
A Father's Affirmation

Dreamer: A man in Alabama

Source: God

Color: Color

Dream Category: Word of Knowledge dream

Dream: I had three dreams over the course of three nights. In my first dream, my dad came to me and told me that he loved me, even if he was not my biological father. The dream was very dark, but my father was illuminated by a spotlight, and there was a pleasant red glow as a backdrop. The second night, I saw my mother and another man (a man whom I recognized but will not name here) in bed together involved in an intimate encounter. The third night, I dreamed about my father again. He was illuminated by a spotlight again and was intent on providing heartfelt reassurance that he loved me no matter what.

Dreamer's Understanding/Interpretation: I felt that these dreams were indicating to me that the man who had raised me was not my biological father, but rather the man in the second dream was my real biological father. I also felt a deep reassurance that the man who had raised me truly loved me.

Author's Spirit-Led Interpretation: This is more of a night vision than a dream, and it was, in fact, a word of knowledge concerning who the dreamer's biological father was.

Impact/Outcome: After the first dream, I called my mother and asked whether my dad (who was no longer living at the time) was, indeed, my biological father. She adamantly denied any possibility that he was not. On the afternoon following the second dream, I called my mother again and talked with her for over forty-five minutes. I explained the dream to her and begged her to tell me whether the second man was actually my biological father. Ultimately, she acknowledged that the second man was, indeed, my birth father, and that only one or two people in the family knew the truth. I was, of course, somewhat distressed, but the final dream the following night brought me deep peace and reassurance that the man whom I had grown up knowing as my father was truly a father to me and that he did love me deeply.

Primary Metaphor(s):

In this particular case, the images in the dream were all literal.

Lesson: It is often difficult to distinguish between a word of knowledge dream and a vision, due to the potential for both to have very literal elements. In the case of a word of knowledge dream, the elements can be interpreted in a way that provides a layer of understanding that is equally valid, but not the direct application of the dream itself. This dream could be interpreted to indicate that the dreamer was deeply loved by his heavenly Father, even in the midst of a potentially uncomfortable family situation. While this interpretation would certainly be applicable, it does not rise to the level of magnitude that the correct understanding of the dream does.

Not only did these dreams communicate the word of knowledge that provided information, but they also ensured that the healing of any potential hurt had been released, even before the pain had an opportunity to arise. It is interesting to note that the assurances and reassurances of love from the man whom the dreamer knew as his father occurred in two separate dreams. It is significant that the healing portion of the dreams was the part that was experienced twice (as with Pharaoh's dream), thus indicating that the love of this father was fixed by God and firmly established as true.

Dream 2:
A Visit from the Surgeon

 (Use the QR code to hear the dreamer give more details about the dream and its significance. If you do not have access to a QR code reader, the Web site associated with this dream is listed in the INDEX.)

Dreamer: A woman in Alabama

Source: God

Color: Color

Dream Category: Healing dream

Dream: While vacationing in Maui, Hawaii, I dreamed that I was in an operating room lying on my back. I opened my eyes (in my dream) and saw a light like what would be used during surgery. A man wearing a surgical mask came into view and asked, "Are you ready?" I said, "Ready for what?" Suddenly I felt an intense pain as a rod went into my breast. The man in the surgical mask then proclaimed, "It is gone, you're healed."

Dreamer's Understanding/Interpretation: I didn't know what to think, but even when I woke, it seemed as if the experience had been real.

Author's Spirit-Led Interpretation: God is about to bring healing to something that has troubled you.

Impact/Outcome: My husband and I had been pastoring a church for about ten years. A few weeks before a planned vacation and sabbatical in Hawaii, I went in for my annual mammogram. Shortly thereafter, I received a letter asking me to come back for a second mammogram for clarification of my results. After the second mammogram, the nurse explained that they would contact me within two weeks by mail. I told her that would not work, because I was leaving town in a few days for a six-week trip. They arranged for a radiologist to review the results immediately, and he found a small area that looked like a cluster of sesame seeds. He informed me that he was somewhat confident the spot was cancerous. When asked how likely it was to be malignant, he responded, "Ninety-five percent sure, but I would need a biopsy and an ultrasound in order to be certain." When he learned that I was leaving town in three days, he insisted that I get a referral and have a biopsy done before leaving for the sabbatical.

After calling my husband, as I waited in the hospital hallway for him to arrive, a spiritual leader we knew walked up and saw me crying. He asked me what was wrong, and I shared my story. He insisted I come with him to see his wife, who happened to be a breast cancer surgeon. He was meeting her there at the hospital for coffee. When I told her the situation, she instructed me to come to her office in an hour's time. My husband arrived, we went to the doctor's office, and she reviewed my test results. She told us that the spots were small and they had been caught early, and she suggested we continue the plans for our trip and take time out to rest. She would do the biopsy when we returned. She told us that we needed to rest and she insisted that we continue with the trip. Then she prayed that God would heal me.

We went on the sabbatical, and I had the dream while we were gone. When we returned from Hawaii six weeks later, I had a stereotactic biopsy (a type of biopsy that involves a rod that is inserted in the breast to remove the tissue sample). Due to an issue with the anesthesia, I felt the same intense pain during the procedure that I had experienced in my dream. Two weeks later, I got the results: The spots were benign. *No cancer!* I am confident that God healed me and removed the cancer through the dream I had in Hawaii.

Primary Metaphor(s):

Surgeon—the Great Physician, God

"It is gone, you are healed"—a prophetic declaration of healing

Lesson: This is an amazing dream in which physical healing was imparted within the dream itself. Notice that there was a physical sensation of pain that lingered even after the dream was complete and the dreamer awoke. This was the first indication that there was a crossover taking place between the spiritual realm, which the dreamer was experiencing within the dream, and the natural realm, in which the dreamer lived.

Given the results of this dream, some might question the author's Spirit-led interpretation as being too generic. However; it is important to remember that God was speaking to the dreamer, and the interpreter's role was simply to help the dreamer understand what God had already said. The interpreter is not responsible for receiving and giving revelation to the dreamer, only for assisting the dreamer to understand what God is already saying to him or her. Unless there is a clear understanding of a more specific interpretation, the interpreter should simply convey what they see and allow God to provide the application of the dream directly to the dreamer. The interpretation given here could have been applied to a physical, spiritual, emotional, or other form of healing, but the dreamer knew immediately that it related to her physical healing, she received comfort, and ultimately, she saw the dream fulfilled in her life.

Dream 3:
A Father's Forgiveness

 (Use the QR code to hear the dreamer give more details about the dream and its significance. If you do not have access to a QR code reader, the Web site associated with this dream is listed in the INDEX.)

Dreamer: A man in West Virginia

Source: God

Color: Color, though the dreamer remembered none

Dream Category: Healing dream

Dream: In this dream, I saw my deceased father standing at the front edge of a walkway on the lawn in front of the home in which I had lived as a child. The walkway itself would have been approximately ten inches to one foot above his feet. I walked up to Dad and embraced him. Dad was too large for me to wrap my arms around, and I had to reach up to embrace him, or at least touch his shoulders. As I embraced Dad, I said to him, "Dad, I love you," and he replied, "I love you, too." As he finished his sentence, we both lifted off the ground and flew up to heaven, just as I had done alone in a dream the previous night. It seemed significant to me that in my dream I had to reach up to embrace Dad. I could only get my hands to the tips of his shoulders and not around him. I was already standing about twelve inches above Dad's feet because of the elevated walkway.

Dreamer's Understanding/Interpretation: After reading a book on dreams, I began to understand the meaning of this dream. It was a dream meant for inner healing, forgiveness, and the restoration of love and respect. Although I had been in an emotional wilderness over this issue, God was granting me the authority to overcome it through the restorative process begun by this dream.

Author's Spirit-Led Interpretation: God is restoring in your heart the love and relationship that you had with your father when you were a child. As He does this, it will lift you up to a new place in your spiritual journey. Although you have been in an emotional wilderness over this issue, God is granting you the authority to overcome it through the restorative process begun in this dream.

Impact/Outcome: About the time I was in the third or fourth grade, the relationship between my dad and me began to deteriorate. By the time I graduated from high school, we had no relationship at all. Dad passed away when I was about twenty-five years old, but although he had passed away, I still had not forgiven him, and my heart was bitter toward him. I did not grasp the full meaning of this dream for almost twenty-seven years. I realized at the time of the dream that I had actually forgiven Dad, and that he had forgiven me. I also realized that my love for Dad had been restored. What I did not realize for all of those years (until I read a book on dreams) was that God had restored the love I had for Dad to the same level that I had had when I was a very young boy, around the age of four or five.

Within a few years of the dream, I found myself in a spiritual battle related to my son and daughter. I am confident that my wife and I would not have had victory in these spiritual battles for our children had I not forgiven my father years earlier. My heart had been full of bitterness that would have influenced my relationship with my own children if God had not taken it away through this dream and restored my love for my dad.

Primary Metaphor(s):

Father—in this case it is a literal figure, although this symbol can often speak of our heavenly Father.

Walkway—a pathway to direct us to a specific destination.

Ten to twelve inches—Ten speaks of wilderness, and twelve is a number that represents authority.

Elevated and flew to heaven—being lifted to a new place in the Spirit

Lesson: This is an amazing dream that addresses inner healing, or emotional healing, that the dreamer needed to experience. The proper interpretation of symbols is essential to understanding a dream, and in this case, recognizing that the father in this dream is literal and does not represent God is vital. While dream dictionaries and similar resources can aid in understanding dream symbols, it is important to remember that the *only* sure way to get it right is to listen to the voice of the Holy Spirit.

Dreams can have both an immediate and a long-term impact on the life of a dreamer. Here, the full understanding of the dream took twenty-seven years to be received, and as such, both the message and the influence of the dream in the dreamer's life was renewed, giving it a lifetime of impact. The dreamer had wandered in a wilderness of bitterness and unforgiveness, but God set him back on a path of authority through restoration and healing that would last throughout his lifetime.

Notice that, in this dream, even when he was on the elevated walkway, the dreamer could not sufficiently reach his father in order to fully embrace him. Reaching up to touch his shoulders reminds us that our primary responsibility is to take the first step when God gives direction, and then let God carry us through the completion of the process.

Dream 4:
A Battle for My Son

 (Use the QR code to hear the dreamer give more details about the dream and its significance. If you do not have access to a QR code reader, the Web site associated with this dream is listed in the INDEX.)

Dreamer: A woman in South Carolina

Source: God

Color: Muted colors

Dream Category: Spiritual warfare dream

Dream: I was at a vacation location with my son and my sister, who had been deeply involved in the occult. My son had been influenced demonically by a toy of some sort that was now talking to him. His behavior had become erratic and not good. At one point, instead of eating, he was under the table rubbing mustard and ketchup into the rug. When I realized this, I told him he needed to clean up the mess. I then walked over to a table of food, looking for fruit or something healthy for him to eat. I saw people at one table getting ice cream cones (the waffle cones that we like). At another table, there was a big cheesecake on the table, but I grabbed a handful of blueberries (although there weren't very many). The plates that people were supposed to use were all dirty. A foreigner started talking to me, and I spoke to him a little. He followed me into the stairwell and asked me in a strong accent about my family trade. I didn't understand what he meant, and then he apologized because Spanish was his first language and he thought that maybe he hadn't spoken the words correctly. I spoke back in Spanish and said we could try to communicate in Spanish, but that I was not completely fluent. He seemed relieved that I spoke Spanish. I then told him he could walk with me. Then it was as if I suddenly was someone else, and I watched that woman almost choke this guy to death out of her anger/frustration over her son and what was going on. The voices from the toy were playing with her son and making him think that it was fun, but really the toy was beginning to torment and control him. The demonic forces were controlling some toys and making them bounce around, and my son thought it was entertaining. They were also tickling him, so that he couldn't rest or take a nap. I finally said, "In Jesus' name, stop tickling him," and a demon spoke through the woman with the occult background in a horrible voice, throwing her around and not wanting to leave . . . but then it finally said, "Okay, I will." I realized then that this was how we were going to need to deal with these forces and that I was going to do whatever necessary to fight for my son's freedom.

Dreamer's Understanding/Interpretation: I understood that this was a warfare dream and that I had actually fought on behalf of my son in the dream. I felt that the Lord was letting me recognize that there were hidden dangers that had affected my son's behavior and influenced him negatively.

Author's Spirit-Led Interpretation: This is a spiritual warfare dream. The enemy brought this dream as an attack against you and to cause fear concerning your son. In the natural realm, some of these attacks may be coming through your children's toys or entertainment that is a part of their lives. Don't try to handle things in your own strength, but do just as you did in the dream: take spiritual authority over the attacks of the enemy and deal with them in that way.

Impact/Outcome: This dream radically affected our family's life. I had thought I was already being careful about the toys and games my son enjoyed, but I then realized that I had been too lenient with some things and that I had allowed an opening for the enemy. We were seeing this manifest in some of his behavior. We removed some of his toys, and he began to improve and grow in his own discernment about what things are not okay. I ultimately wrote about this dream and what I had learned in my blog so that perhaps it would also help other people.

Primary Metaphor(s):

Vacation place—a place where one would expect to rest

Rubbing mustard and ketchup—rebellion, damaging activities

Not eating/looking for healthy food—a lack of spiritual nourishment and knowledge that it is needed

Foreigner—someone/something unfamiliar

Lesson: This is a spiritual warfare dream sent by the enemy. It would be easy to assume that it should simply be ignored; however, when a Spirit-led interpretation is applied to any dream, there is always something that we can learn and gain life from. In this case, the Lord allowed this dream in order for the dreamer's attention to be called to an area of spiritual attack against her family that was occurring outside of the dream.

An important foundational principle relating to how we deal with spiritual warfare dreams can also be gleaned from this dream. It is important that we not react to the dream, but instead that we respond in a godly fashion. Here, the dreamer "turns into someone else" as she deals with those around her who might have had wisdom, but who were not able to communicate it easily. Recognizing this, she then steps back and exercises spiritual authority over the attack to bring it to an end.

Finally, it is important to realize that the dream realm is a spiritual realm. We can speak to the adversaries in our dreams and take authority over them. While there is no atmosphere present through which the vibrations created from our vocal cords can travel, we can still take authority in our spirit or respond in a fashion that conveys the spiritual authority we carry. By taking authority in our spiritual warfare dreams, not only do we keep them from recurring and draining us, but we also set a tone for how the attacks can be overcome in our waking lives.

Dream 5:
God Speaks

Dreamer: Ashley Taylor[1], a woman in Alabama, with the dream recounted by her brother

Source: God

Color: Color

Dream Category: Warning dream

Dream: In my dream, Jesus came and woke me up. He told me that He wanted to talk to me, and we just talked for a while. After a period of time, Jesus told me that He had been with me and saved me many, many times, but that my time was up at the rehabilitation center and it was important for me to move on. He said that it was time to step up and do the right thing in my life, because He was going to let me make some choices for myself. Then He explained that if I did drugs again, I would die.

Dreamer's Understanding/Interpretation: Without an interpretation, this dream frightened the dreamer and caused her to wonder whether or not she was crazy, because it seemed so real. However, the peacefulness of the conversation stood out to her.

---

[1] This is the only dream included in this book in which the dreamer is identified by name. This is done in Ashley's case at the request of her family, in the hope that her story might help to save the life of another who may one day find themselves in a similar situation.

Author's Spirit-Led Interpretation: The Lord is warning you that it is time to make a major change in your life and deal with the issues that have plagued you for some time. This is a serious warning, and it will have significant consequences if it is not heeded.

Impact/Outcome: The dreamer had been addicted to drugs and had gotten "clean" through rehabilitation at the Love Lady Center in Birmingham, Alabama. As is the case in the lives of many addicts, there were times of struggle, and she had relapsed several times. The dreamer overdosed on heroine the following week after this dream and died. As her brother recounted the dream, he also indicated that his sister had shared something that only God could have known before it happened, and as a result, it caused him to believe that God does indeed speak through dreams.

Primary Metaphor(s):

Conversation with Jesus—prophetic insight into the dreamer's life

Lesson: Although the outcome of this dream is unlike any other reported in this book, and ultimately is tragic in nature, it conveys perhaps one of the greatest lessons that can be learned from *Dream Stories*. God desires to speak to His children, and one of the ways He does this is through dreams. It is essential that we begin to believe that God does speak, and that when He does, we *must* listen to what He is telling us.

The warning in this dream is very direct and needs little interpretation. When revelation is given in such a direct way, it carries with it a very high level of accountability. There was a responsibility given in this dream for the dreamer to obey the direction and receive the encouragement that she could overcome the challenge of her addiction. Although the dreamer failed to heed this warning, her tragic death becomes a powerful lesson for those around her and for those who hear her story.

Dream 6:
Cutting Out My Tongue

 *(Use the QR code to hear the dreamer give more details about the dream and its significance. If you do not have access to a QR code reader, the Web site associated with this dream is listed in the INDEX.)*

Dreamer: A man in Alabama

Source: God

Color: Vivid color

Dream Category: Deliverance dream

Dream: I dreamed that I was in an old house. As I walked through the house, I entered a room where a beautiful woman dressed in white with radiant golden hair was waiting. I walked up to the woman and stood directly in front of her, but I could not describe her in any more detail. As I stood there, she looked at me intently, as if she was looking inside of me. In that moment, I knew that she wanted me to stick out my tongue. In response, I stuck my tongue out slightly, and she grabbed it and pulled it out a little more. Next, she took a sword from her side and cut my tongue off. It was not painful, but it was startling. After standing there a few more minutes, I knew that she wanted me to stick my tongue out again. This time she grabbed it and pulled. It seemed as if she pulled it out a very great distance. She then took the sword and cut it off a second time. Again, it was not painful, but still shocking. I knew that even though she had cut my tongue out twice, it was still there. When I awoke the next morning, my wife told me that twice during the night I had shaken so violently in the bed that it had roused her from sleep.

Dreamer's Understanding/Interpretation: When I had the dream, I knew that it meant that something within me was changing and that I was being released. My friend and mentor told me that this was an encounter with an angel and that God was setting me free from something that had hindered my ability to communicate.

Author's Spirit-Led Interpretation: God is removing something that has inhibited your ability to communicate what you have inside of you.

Impact/Outcome: For years prior to this dream, I had had recurring dreams that I had something in my mouth that I could not get out. In various dreams, it might be bubble gum, cotton candy, caramel, or any of several other things. After this dream, I never had that recurring dream again. I had entered the ministry shortly before the dream, and I was a new pastor. I had been struggling to communicate the spiritual truths that God showed me, but from the time of this dream forward, I gained a new freedom of expression and my ability to speak, preach, and teach increased dramatically.

Primary Metaphor(s):

Old house—dreamer's life

Woman in white—an angel

Tongue—the capacity to speak

Sword—something that is cutting (as in cutting words); in this case it indicates a beneficial cutting away of that which had been a hindrance

Lesson: This dream involves a literal angelic visitation. Often people think that encountering a spiritual being only takes place when a person is awake and cognitive of their surroundings; however, this is not always the case. Throughout the Scriptures, angelic visitations occurred both during waking moments (for example, see 1 Kings 19 and Matthew 28:2) and during dreams (for example, see Matthew 1:20, 2:13, and 2:19). Spiritual beings in dreams can often (though not always) be identified when the dreamer remembers the individual vividly, but the dreamer often cannot describe any particular facial features. For this reason, spiritual beings in dreams are often called "faceless people."

Because the dreamer had been set free from an ungodly hindrance, this encounter is described as a deliverance dream. In this case, the dream also involved a physical manifestation in the waking world of the deliverance that was taking place in the dream. The dreamer's spouse recounted waking up and finding the dreamer violently shaking in the bed twice during the night—presumably each time the angel cut the dreamer's tongue.

Dream 7:
Dwelling on My Loss

Dreamer: A man in West Virginia

Source: Soul

Color: Muted colors

Dream Category: Soul dream

Dream: In my dream, my girlfriend (a girl with whom I had been obsessed in high school) and I had broken up, and she quickly moved on and got married to someone else. I was getting ready to go to a prom/high school reunion event. My mother told me that my old girlfriend would not be at the event. She said that her new husband was a rock star and that they would be on tour at that time. I thought about this for a time in the dream, and I had a sense of lost hope. I remembered how I had stopped talking to her for a period of time after our breakup. I felt sad that she had moved on. I was only going to the event because I had thought that I would run into her again, so I decided that I wouldn't go. I was driving my current car, a silver Mustang, in the dream, and I was back in my hometown. I thought about driving by her old house, but then I decided against it.

Dreamer's Understanding/Interpretation: This dream caused me to have regret for how I had behaved in real life.

Author's Spirit-Led Interpretation: This is a soul dream that is arising from things on which you are dwelling on and dealing with in your life. God wants you to move beyond your past and into your destiny. He is ready for you to move quickly into a powerful new purpose.

Impact/Outcome: The dreamer was left with tremendous feelings of loss, regret, and nostalgia.

Primary Metaphor(s):

High school girlfriend—soulish desire for an old relationship

Mother—the Holy Spirit, who was seeking to guide the dreamer away from this soulish desire

Silver—redemption

Mustang automobile—powerful purpose or destiny

Lesson: Dreams that originate in our souls are commonly an expression of our personal desires coming forth in our dreams. While these dreams do not provide direction from the Lord, it is important to note that when they are understood correctly, they can help identify issues that need to be dealt with, and, as in this case, the Lord can insert His wisdom and direction into the dreams if we are willing to see it. This type of dream can be considered a form of self-reflection when it is properly understood.

Notice how the dreamer awakens from this dream with a deep sense of loss and regret. This is not a positive impact from the dream itself; however, even a dream that originates from our own souls can have a positive impact when a godly interpretation is provided and the dream is understood for what it is. After the interpretation is made known to the dreamer, he or she now has a choice to continue in the regret that the dream seemed to stir up, or accept the alternative plan that the Lord identifies through the interpretation. If they do so, they can then move forward with a new sense of purpose, leaving the past behind and stepping forward into their destiny in the Lord.

Dream Stories by Michael B. French

Page | 92

Dream 8:
Imprisoned

Dreamer: An obnoxious drunk man in Poland[24]

Source: The enemy

Color: Black and white

Dream Category: Dark dream

Dream: I dreamed that I was in a prison. I was locked up, and it was dark and gloomy. I had been locked away in the prison for some time. Even though I was a prisoner, I still had a sword, and when men would come into my cell, I would stab them and kill them. I enjoyed every bit of it.

Dreamer's Understanding/Interpretation: The dreamer did not even know a dream could be interpreted.

Author's Spirit-Led Interpretation: This dream is about the dreamer's life. Something happened to you at a very young age that put you on a path of hatred, anger, and resentment. It has locked you in a prison of darkness. You have been given a gift by God to give life to men rather than death.

Impact/Outcome: The dreamer began to cry, and the team led him to the Lord. He told the minister that he and his friend had intended to get even more drunk that night and go break into houses. He explained how they had already decided to harm or kill anyone who was home. Because of this encounter, he and his friend decided not to carry out their plan.

Primary Metaphor(s):

Prison—a place of captivity

Stabbing and killing—anger, rage, hatred

Lesson: One of the most important lessons that can be learned from encounters with dark dreams from the enemy is that they will almost certainly present a lie. While these dreams do not come from God, they can still be used by God to impact the life of the dreamer. By "flipping" the dream—looking for the opposite of what the enemy's message was intended to convey—the way in which God sees the dreamer will often be revealed. This dreamer was imprisoned by anger and hatred, but it was not who he was created to be. A spiritual interpretation to a demonically inspired dream brought hope to the dreamer and changed the course of his life. Often the interpretation of dark dreams will involve an element of dream interpretation mixed with an element of prophetic revelation. Here, the individual who interpreted the dream was able to understand its negative meaning, but he was also able to provide hope. The interpretation required the interpreter to be able to hear God's voice as He prophetically revealed His plan and purpose for the dreamer's life, as opposed to what the enemy had thrust upon him.

The enemy wanted to keep the dreamer in prison, yet it is clear that God desired him to be free. The anger, rage, and hatred that the dreamer enjoyed in the dream was presented in a fashion intended to rob him of hope for any change in his life. By identifying the hope that God offered, speaking to the dreamer in love, and helping him to see a way out of the bondage that had held him captive, a life-giving interpretation came forth, even though the dream was intended for evil.

Dream 9:
Finding the Ring

Dreamer: A woman in Alabama

Source: God

Color: Color

Dream Category: Word of Knowledge dream

Dream: I dreamed that I told my sister to go look in her closet for a diamond ring that she had lost. I told her that it was in a black purse. She argued with me that the ring was not in the closet. I insisted that she needed to go and look anyway, then I woke up.

Dreamer's Understanding/Interpretation: I felt like my sister's missing diamond ring might be in a purse in her closet.

Author's Spirit-Led Interpretation: Tell your sister to look in a purse in her closet for her missing ring.

Impact/Outcome: My sister had just shared with me that she had been keeping a very expensive diamond ring for a friend and that when she moved to her new home, it turned up missing. She was concerned that someone had stolen the ring, and she was very upset. I had the dream that afternoon while taking a nap. When I awoke, I called my sister to tell her the dream, and she insisted that the ring could not be in her closet and that she did not have a black purse. I suggested that she look anyway, and when she did she found the ring exactly as she had in the dream.

Primary Metaphor(s):

Closet—hidden

Ring—often refers to a covenant, but it was literal in this case

Lesson: Coming so quickly after the telephone conversation with her sister, this dream needed very little interpretation. A word of knowledge provides a solution to a particular problem or gives the answer to a question, and that is exactly what this dream did. The greatest lesson from this dream is conveyed when we understand how important it can be to follow through with what we learn from a dream. This dream gave the dreamer the ability to convey prophetic information in a safe way and brought the benefit of that revelation to life not only for the dreamer, but also for her sister.

It would have been easy for the dreamer to ignore this dream and assume that it was nothing more than an internal expression of her outward concern for her sister and the predicament in which she found herself. Consider how easy it would have been to ignore what God was saying and take no action on the dream whatsoever. By learning to value all dreams and to trust our heavenly Father to both provide the interpretation and reveal the application of it, there was a tremendous opportunity for the dreamer's faith to be increased and for the sister's dilemma to be resolved.

Dream 10:
Encountering Jesus at a Coffee Shop

Dreamer: A woman in Minnesota

Source: God

Color: Muted (as reported by the dreamer), but actually normal color

Dream Category: Courage dream

Dream: I enter a coffee shop, and to my left are a couple of men at a small table. They are dressed in shirts and slacks/jeans. I glance in the direction of the man facing me—he has a friendly face and curly black hair, with a Mediterranean look about him. Our eyes meet, and I casually greet him as I move toward the counter. I get my coffee and go out the door. The man with the curly black hair catches up to me, puts his arm around my shoulder, and says, "You showed courage today!" With his arm still around my shoulder, we continue walking toward a wall where the other man is now standing, waiting for us. His face is not distinguishable. As we come up to him, the dream ends.

Dreamer's Understanding/Interpretation: I understood the Mediterranean-looking man in this dream to be Jesus, communicating to me through the dream and encouraging me.

Author's Spirit-Led Interpretation: The Lord is pleased with you as you have stepped out in faith, and He wants you to continue to walk with Him in that courage so that you may have an impact on other lives around you.

Impact/Outcome: This dream came the night after I attended a Minnesota prayer breakfast as an intercessor, and I was very much a "green horn." We had waited for people to come up for prayer after the event, but no one came, so I asked permission to see if anyone who was leaving wanted prayer. This was very difficult for me to do, but when I did, I was able to pray for a young man and his family. When the Lord asks me to do something now, even if I dread it and want to decline, I remember this dream and I try to step out in faith.

Primary Metaphor(s):

Man with friendly face—the Lord

Arm around shoulder/continued walking—God will be with you as you keep moving forward

Lesson: In this case, when the dreamer was asked whether there was color in the dream, she replied that it seemed muted. However, as she recounted the dream, and she was asked if any colors stood out, she specifically mentioned that "it was a bright, sunny day." While color is an indicator of whether a dream comes from God, dreamers' interpretations of the colors in their dreams can vary based upon their own experiences. A dream can be described as muted, but when it is examined more carefully, as in this case, the colors in the dream may not actually be muted, but rather just normal. If a person is accustomed to dreaming in vivid color, and then he or she has a dream in normal color, it may seem muted at the time. If a person is accustomed to dreaming in black and white, and then he or she has a dream with muted colors, it may seem vivid. Even when the dreamer describes the color of their dream, it is important to hear what the Holy Spirit has to say about where the dream originates.

Dream 11:
John Paul Jackson Takes a Bite of Eggs

 *(Use the QR code to hear the dreamer give more details about the dream and its significance. If you do not have access to a QR code reader, the Web site associated with this dream is listed in the INDEX.)*

Dreamer: A woman in Georgia

Source: God

Color: Color

Dream Category: Prophetic dream

Dream: I dreamed that I was at a picnic area outside on a beautiful day. There were long, rectangular tables, and I was eating breakfast with a group of people while John Paul Jackson was standing before the group teaching. John Paul walked over to my table and took a bite of my eggs with a fork.

Dreamer's Understanding/Interpretation: The dream was revealing that John Paul Jackson would use a question I had asked for his YouTube video entitled *Colors in Dreams*.

Author's Spirit-Led Interpretation: God is revealing that you have something that will be nourishing to the prophetic community around you.

Impact/Outcome: This dream showed me that God will show us all things. When I saw the video (https://www.youtube.com/watch?v=4QY4U_ATv8k), I realized that my dream had indeed revealed that John Paul Jackson would use my question to help him to teach others. This dream also caused me to realize how important it is to keep track of all of my dreams, no matter how silly they may seem.

Primary Metaphor(s):

Eggs—spiritual food

John Paul Jackson—prophetic ministry

Lesson: While the simple Spirit-led interpretation of this dream does not indicate the specific prophetic nature of the dream, it does provide a general prophetic word. The dream broadly prophesies to the dreamer that, even as she is learning to sustain herself (by eating the eggs), she has value to offer to others that will be noticed and shared. This is precisely what happened when John Paul Jackson drew from her question to teach on color in his video, and that specific prophetic fulfillment of the dream gave the dreamer confidence that the general prophetic impartation of the dream was also valid for her life.

Dream 12:
Airplane Crash into the Ocean

 *(Use the QR code to hear the dreamer give more details about the dream and its significance. If you do not have access to a QR code reader, the Web site associated with this dream is listed in the INDEX.)*

Dreamer: A woman in Georgia

Source: God

Color: Color

Dream Category: Correction dream

Dream: This was a recurring dream of mine for several years. I was on a 747 jet, and I saw a young boy sitting nearby. I had a very tiny newborn baby in my purse, and I could see palm trees in the window as we flew over the ocean. The plane crashed into the ocean. The door opened to the plane when it hit the bottom, and I could see a light shining through the door, leading the way up to the top of the water. I grabbed my purse with the tiny baby and followed the light to the top of the ocean and began swimming toward an island. The blue color of the ocean brought peace, even though I had just been in a plane crash. When I got to the shore, there were some Africans wearing little cloths, and they took my purse and started running away. I screamed, "There's a baby in the purse!" I did not want them to hurt the baby.

Dreamer's Understanding/Interpretation: Two different people interpreted this dream as related to my finances, but I couldn't understand why at first. The interpretation indicated that there was an unsanctified giving connected to my finances.

Author's Spirit-Led Interpretation: God has given you financial gifts that can have tremendous impact in the Kingdom of God, but it is not yet mature. The enemy's plan is to steal the resources God has given you by using those who seem to be in need, but who actually only want to take what you have. Even though things may crash all around you, God is showing you the way of escape.

Impact/Outcome: Before I understood the interpretation, this dream brought fear, and I would not get on an airplane for many years because I thought the interpretation was literal. I knew I was a giver, but I could not figure out how the interpretation I had been given could be true, until my husband lost his job a few years later. I then realized how much I had given away to others (through unsanctified "mercy giving"). After this, I reevaluated what I was doing based upon the dream and the wisdom it had brought. I learned the importance of saving for the future and how unsanctified "mercy giving" can crash your finances.

Primary Metaphor(s):

Baby—new/immature gift

Purse—often indicates favor, but in this case, it referred to the dreamer's finances

Door open/light shining in—a way of escape

Lesson: Remember that soulish interpretations can result in the life of a spiritual dream being lost, just as this dream caused fear until a Spirit-led interpretation was received and understood. Spiritual interpretations provide hope. The hope was always there in the dream (the blue water caused the dreamer to feel peace, even though she had just been in a plane crash, even before the dream was properly interpreted), but the Spirit interpretation was needed to release the meaning. This was a gentle way of correcting how the dreamer was using her gift. Notice that even though some of what the enemy had planned had been able to impact the dreamer's life, God still used the dream to teach the dreamer and to help bring her "baby" to a new level of maturity.

Dream 13
Depression Gone

Dreamer: A woman in Alabama

Source: God

Color: Color

Dream Category: Healing dream

Dream: I was riding in a black car that broke down on the side of the road. I was so disgusted and angry. After a while, my mom came along. She bumped into my car and pushed it over the embankment. "Get in," she said. She was driving a beautiful, shiny red car. I got in, and we drove away laughing.

Dreamer's Understanding/Interpretation: I had lost both my mom and my dad in March of 2014, and I had been struggling with dark depression, even though I knew both of them were with Jesus. I know the black car represented the state I was in. The red car represented the anointing of the Holy Spirit. After meditating in prayer about the dream, the depression left and my joy returned.

Author's Spirit-Led Interpretation: This dream is about the place of emotional discomfort you are in on your journey through life. God is wanting you to leave that place behind and move forward with joy into a new level of anointing.

Impact/Outcome: This dream helped to return me to a place of joy. I laugh now when I think about the dream, and while I still miss my parents terribly, my thoughts are no longer dark.

Primary Metaphor(s):

Cars—ministry or life (in this case, the dreamer's life journey)

Black—darkness, death

Bumping car over embankment—time to leave it behind and let go

Lesson: Emotions felt in a dream often help with understanding the interpretation, but they can also be an indication of the state of mind of the dreamer. In this case, the emotional responses in the dream—disgust and anger—transform into joy and laughter, indicating the change that God wants to bring about in the dreamer's state of being. Notice that while the dreamer's mother (who had passed away) was in the dream, the Spirit-led interpretation did not address her presence in the dream. While in this case, the dreamer understood the dream without an outside interpretation, had she received the Spirit-led interpretation, she would have known it related to her mother based upon her own experiences and emotional state. Keep in mind that dreamers generally already know what they are going through and an interpretation from another person does not have to identify every detail in order for the dreamer to understand its full meaning.

Dream 14:
I'm in Charge Here!

 (Use the QR code to hear the dreamer give more details about the dream and its significance. If you do not have access to a QR code reader, the Web site associated with this dream is listed in the INDEX.)

Dreamer: A male pastor in England

Source: God

Color: Color

Dream Category: Warning dream

Dream: In my dream, my wife and I were going up some stairs into an upper room, where there were plenty of people whom I seemed to know, even though I could not see their faces. They were people from our church. The room was unusual, because the ceiling was under a mansard roof. (Somehow, I knew it had a mansard roof: a roof that has four sloping sides, each of which becomes steeper halfway down.) The only other feature in the room was a window, nine feet up from the floor, through which all I could see was blue sky. Then my eyes were drawn to the ceiling immediately above me, where there was a trapdoor that led into the roof space. The panel of the trapdoor had been moved aside, and out of the trapdoor came a huge python snake. It was brown with big, bright yellow spots all over it. As it came farther down into the room, maybe a few feet, I could see that it was as thick as my upper leg. *Big!* I knew it was not going to attack anyone, but as I looked into its eyes, I saw what is referred to in Proverbs 6:17 as one of the "things the Lord hates": haughty eyes. These were the haughtiest eyes I had ever seen, and my blood began to run cold as I realized that the python was not going to physically harm anyone. He was merely checking to see that he was still in control. Then I woke up.

Dreamer's Understanding/Interpretation: My wife and I knew what the symbols meant, but we could not find any hope in the dream at first. The interpretation was that our church was either already under the control, or would soon be under the control, of a python spirit (a leviathan spirit), which we knew was not only a lying spirit but also one that wanted to squeeze the prophetic life out of our church and shut down any revelation from God. It was working through a small group of people (we knew who they were) who were intellectually opposed to divine revelation and of a more humanistic than spiritual persuasion, driven by fear.

Author's Spirit-Led Interpretation: This dream is a warning that you and your church need to stay alert to a spiritual attack that will operate through fear and a humanistic mindset. Its purpose is to choke the life out of any prophetic revelation in your church. The feeling of superiority in those who are affected by this spiritual assault will cause them to operate as though they are above everyone else and better in control of what is going on.

Impact/Outcome: The dream caused me to do a great deal of study on the leviathan/python spirit and to seek out others to help me understand the interpretation of the dream. For about six months, I was obsessed with searching for hope in the dream. This ultimately made me more determined than ever to pursue prophetic things and divine revelation in our church.

I shared the dream with John Paul Jackson, an internationally known revelation minister, because I needed to know how to deal with this warning. He prophetically explained that as we continued to worship the Lord, preach the truth, encourage divine revelation, and continue in Kingdom work, those who were opposed or fearful to what was going on would ultimately leave the church (they did); the floor would rise, and we would all be able to see through the window and fulfill the prophecies and visions that the Lord had given to us.

Primary Metaphor(s):

Window—vision, revelation

Snake—lies; pythons are constrictors, which squeeze the life out of their prey

Brown—in this case, the color brown is negative and represents humanism

Yellow—in this case, the color yellow is negative and represents fear

Lesson: Warning dreams do not always provide the solution as much as they identify the problem. The dreamer responded in the most appropriate way possible: by seeking further understanding and digging into the Word of God to find the needed answers. As was the case in this dream, it can also be very helpful to seek out others who have deeper revelation to help you understand the response for which dreams sometimes call. Simply knowing the interpretation to this dream was not enough; it required action and a response in order for the dreamer to heed the warning (just as Pharaoh had to act on his dream of the wheat and the cows found in Genesis 41).

It should be noted that John Paul Jackson's insight was not a further interpretation of the dream, but a prophetic response providing a solution for the warning that had already been given in the dream.

Dream 15:
Will 1 Sink?

 (Use the QR code to hear the dreamer give more details about the dream and its significance. If you do not have access to a QR code reader, the Web site associated with this dream is listed in the INDEX.)

Dreamer: A woman in England

Source: God

Color: Color

Dream Category: Calling dream

Dream: I had this dream in the fall of 2003. I was in my own little yellow submarine under the sea but near the shore. Suddenly the submarine broke through the surface of the water, and all I could see was the huge prow of a large white ocean liner. I thought it might run into me because it was so close.

Dreamer's   Understanding/Interpretation: I misinterpreted the dream. I had cancer in the spring of 2003, and so I thought this was a dream about my upcoming death. I knew nothing about dream interpretation at that time.

Author's Spirit-Led Interpretation: The work that you have been functioning in has been hidden, but it is soon going to become visible suddenly and be noticed by a large ministry.

Impact/Outcome: The misinterpretation caused me to have tremendous anxiety that I was going to die. But when the dream was properly interpreted, the impact was great in my life, giving me hope and excitement. Sometime thereafter, the ministry that my husband and I were conducting was noticed, and we were called upon to work together with a much larger ministry to establish a training center in the United Kingdom and expand the work it was doing to other parts of Europe, as well.

Primary Metaphor(s):

Submarine—a ministry that operates hidden beneath the surface

Yellow—fear, gifts, or hope

Ocean liner—a large ministry with widespread impact

Lesson: This dream is a clear illustration of a soulish interpretation to a Spirit-given dream resulting in little or no fruit. It is possible to be totally wrong in one's interpretation of the meaning of a dream and thus operate in fear or confusion until the correct interpretation is provided. Here, the dreamer misinterpreted the dream out of fear. Nowhere in the dream did the ocean liner ever strike the submarine, and it should not be assumed that it would just because it was so close. Instead, the closeness of the ship related to the nearness of God to what the dreamer was doing. When a true spiritual interpretation was finally provided, the value of this dream came forth and was life-changing for the dreamer.

Also, notice that while the initial misinterpretation of the dream caused fear, when the mind of Christ was put on, in order to see the dream as it was intended, it brought hope. The yellow color of the submarine had potential for either a positive or negative meaning in this dream. Yellow could relate either to fear or to hope, depending upon the context of the dream. The submarine (something that is normally hidden beneath the surface) was breaking through and becoming visible in the dream. This context indicates that the dreamer's gifts were about to be noticed, and thus the Spirit-led interpretation of the color yellow was dependent upon the context of the dream.

Dream Stories by Michael B. French

Dream 16:
Where Do the Righteous Run?

Dreamer: A woman in Alabama

Source: God

Color: Color

Dream Category: Courage dream

Dream: I'm in a room at the top of a tall concrete building/tower. There are three large windows in the room, each one facing a different direction: south, west, and north. I can see multiple (three or more) tornadoes fingering down through each window. I turn to the door behind me (east), and I rush out into the lobby/reception area to instruct the staff to get the children down to the lowest level of the building immediately (to protect them). Once the students have made it down to safety, I turn toward the door to the reception area, board the elevator, and go down to join them. However, my way is blocked; there are large boxes in my way, and the time is too short. There is an unknown person to my left who is with me. I turn to him and say, "Brace yourself (between the boxes, as I do the same). We're going to take a hit!" I'm braced and waiting, waiting . . . but there is no hit?!? Then I stand up, with a strange understanding, and say, "It's okay. It's not going to hit here." Then I woke up. This is the *only* time in my life when I've ever woken up with an immediate scripture passage on my lips or in my mind: "The name of the LORD is a strong tower; the righteous man runs into it and is safe" (Proverbs 18:10, ESV).

Dreamer's Understanding/Interpretation: I felt this dream was a reminder that, as I see storms approach, I should not allow myself to be moved by fear or anything other than the Lord. The storms may come from all different directions, and they may look terrifying and intimidating, but my safety is secure in the Lord. I should not leave my post.

Author's Spirit-Led Interpretation: This is a dream encouraging you that your shelter is in the Lord and that you do not have to fear the storms that come against you.

Impact/Outcome: This dream caused me to realize how much God cares about me. He gave me a dream and a scripture verse to remind me to be strong and not to fear. Years later, on April 27, 2011, my husband and I awoke to the sound of tornado sirens. [Author's note: This was one of the largest and deadliest tornado outbreaks ever recorded, with 355 confirmed tornadoes. The dreamer's home state of Alabama was one of the hardest hit areas.] As we made our way down to the basement, the Holy Spirit stopped me in my tracks and said, "Speak, child!" I began to speak to the storm. We lost five trees, and the screens were ripped off of our porch, but that was the extent of the damage we suffered. I felt that this was one of the storms that I had seen in my dream, and I knew that God would be there through any other storms I would face in my lifetime.

Primary Metaphor(s):

Tornadoes—storms either literal or symbolic of spiritual attacks

Brace yourself—get ready

No hit—the Lord's protection

Lesson: This is a courage dream, because it is intended to instill courage in the dreamer to face the circumstances that are coming. Interpreting this dream in a short, general way allows the Holy Spirit to provide the insight as to whether the storms in the dream represent attacks from the enemy or natural storms. It is possible for a tornado in a dream to represent physical, spiritual, mental, or emotional attacks or trials. In this case, the dream does not provide specific information as to whether the storms would be natural or spiritual in their nature, and unless the Holy Spirit makes this clear, it is best not to assume that one or the other is true.

It is not uncommon for dreams to have layers of meaning, and such is the case in this particular instance. After the events of April 27, 2011, it became clear that this dream related to those events and thereby was referring to natural storms. It was this dream that actually gave the dreamer the courage to remember that she would be okay during this terrible tornado outbreak. However, stopping there would not have provided a complete understanding of the dream's meaning. The physical protection provided by the Lord on April 27 also provided a natural confirmation of the further meaning of the dream: that the dreamer could trust the Lord to shelter her during any other types of attack and trials that she would face on her journey through life, because the Lord is, indeed, the dreamer's strong tower, where she can be safe.

Dream 17: Decision

Dreamer: A man in Mississippi

Source: God

Color: Color

Dream Category: Self-condition dream

Dream: I was sitting at the peak of a huge arch, similar to the Saint Louis Arch, looking out over the countryside from a couple hundred feet above the ground. It was a beautiful sight, and I was very comfortable sitting there. There were green fields and farms below. I did not want to leave. It had been a long, hard climb up to this perch, and I just wanted to enjoy myself there, but I realized I had to get back to the ground. The question was, Did I go back down the way I had come up, or should I go down the other side of the arch? I knew what it was like where I had come from and what the climb was like. If I chose to go down the other side, I did not know what the descent would be like or even where I would end up. Eventually, I made the decision to go down the other side and I immediately awoke.

Dreamer's Understanding/Interpretation: The Lord was showing me in the dream that I had a major decision to make: I could go back the way I had come and land to a safe place, or I could step out in a new direction, even though I did not know what would happen or where I would end up.

Author's Spirit-Led Interpretation: This dream is about changing the way you approach life. It is time to move into a place of real growth and take a risk, leaving behind the comfort of what you have known to press forward into what lies ahead.

Impact/Outcome: After making the decision to take the new path in the dream, I began to make similar decisions in my life, forgoing the safe paths and reaching out to the new and different paths set before me.

Primary Metaphor(s):

Green fields and farms—places where things grow

Arch—the decision will have an overarching impact on every area of your life

Choice of direction—decision needing to be made

Lesson: Remember that self-condition dreams don't simply show us where we are, but they also help us to recognize decisions that need to be made in our lives. In this case, the dreamer is being reminded that he has a part to play in choosing how he lives his life. and that moving into a place of fruitfulness may not always be the easiest choice to make. The choice made in a dream often helps the dreamer by making his or her choices in life easier to decide upon and pursue.

John Wimber, founder of The Vineyard churches, once said, "Faith is spelled *R-I-S-K*." Notice how the risk associated with going down the unknown side of the arch in this dream becomes a metaphor for faith. This is an illustration of how the symbols in dreams can be understood both through their natural purpose (the new direction carried with it unknown qualities that would cause the dreamer to end up in a place he had not experienced before) or through colloquialisms and common usage (the risk associated with taking the unknown path requires faith to go into the new places that God is drawing the dreamer to go).

Dream Stories by Michael B. French

Dream 18:
A Warning for His Daughter

Dreamer: A woman in Alabama

Source: God

Color: Color

Dream Category: Courage dream

Dream: We were on a huge cruise ship, below the main deck. The Holy Spirit spoke to me and told me that the ship was about to make a 180-degree turn, but that we would have to go underwater for the ship to make this turnaround. He physically showed me in my dream the pressure I would feel while it was underwater, but that we would come back safely. I agreed and braced myself. In my dream, I could feel everything, even going underwater and experiencing the pressure. The ship came back up like the Holy Spirit had promised, and I remember seeing a beautiful blue sky and a brilliant sun. The ship docked at an island in the middle of the ocean. People were filing out of the ship onto the island. They were headed toward a church there. When we went in, I went with our kids to children's church, and my husband went straight toward the sanctuary.

Dreamer's Understanding/Interpretation: I felt the dream identified a path that I was on and the need for a major shift to take place in my life. I knew from the brightness of the sun and the clarity of the blue sky that I could overcome the pressure it would take to make that shift.

Author's Spirit-Led Interpretation: Your life is intended to have a major impact on those around you, but something needs to change in order for that to happen. The Lord is encouraging you that the difficulty it takes to make the turnaround you need to make will be worth it in the end. After this shift, the impact your life will have on your children's lives will be increased.

Impact/Outcome: This dream marked a major turning point in my life. After the dream, my husband and I began to recognize a major shift in our lives. We walked into a time of wilderness that lasted three years and was one of the darkest times I had ever experienced, but I remembered that I would be okay because of what the Holy Spirit had told me in the dream. God used that time to show me how legalistic I had become, and to help me understand the fullness of His love and grace. God brought us out of that dark period, just like He had promised, but I don't think I could have gone through what it took if it hadn't been for what He had previously showed me in this dream.

Primary Metaphor(s):

Cruise ship—dreamer's life/ministry that has a major impact

180-degree turn—you are going in the wrong direction

Pressure—trial or difficulty

Blue sky—favor after the course correction

Lesson: This dream helps to provide understanding of how dreams and visions can overlap (even with the more open-ended definitions that are being used in this book). Notice that this dream contains elements that need to be interpreted (as a dream) and elements that do not (as a vision). The metaphors in this dream clearly indicate the need for a change, but the Holy Spirit also spoke a direct word and clearly showed the dreamer things using these metaphors. The promise that the dreamer could make it through the pressure needs no interpretation. The metaphors in this dream only help to assist the dreamer in understanding to what the pressure will be related and why it would be worth it in the end.

The symbols and imagery of dreams are not limited to visual representations. It is significant in this dream that the pressure associated with the ship going under the water was literally felt in the dream. The use of this physical sensation is also a metaphor that can be interpreted. Here, the physical pressure of the water is symbolic of the spiritual, mental, and emotional pressure that would be felt as a result of the course correction that needed to be made in the dreamer's life. It is important that when seeking to comprehend a dream, we do not limit the Holy Spirit to providing only understanding of the visual symbolism, but that we also allow Him to provide explanations for sounds, smells, tastes, feelings (both emotional and physical), and more.

Dream 19:
Don't Give Up

 (Use the QR code to hear the dreamer give more details about the dream and its significance. If you do not have access to a QR code reader, the Web site associated with this dream is listed in the INDEX.)

Dreamer: A woman in Alabama

Source: The enemy, but God intervenes

Color: Muted colors with a single, bright-colored element

Dream Category: Courage dream

Dream: In my dream, I was living in a house that was built into a mountain. The back door of the kitchen opened into a cave-like passage within the mountain. There was a treasure in the mountain, and I wanted to get it. I saw it one time in the dream, and it looked like something you would see in an old pirate movie. Guarding the treasure were many crocodiles. There were many people at the beginning of the dream who were trying to help me get to my treasure, but it was dangerous and I knew that people could get hurt. I remember having to call the medics for one man who sustained a serious arm wound. Then there came a giant crocodile that ate all the other crocodiles. At this point, I was alone, except for one unseen person who was going to help me face the single giant crocodile. Just as I was opening the back door to face the crocodile, I woke up. I did not recognize anyone in the dream, but I remember that the tablecloth in kitchen was red-and-white checked.

Dreamer's Understanding/Interpretation: I felt that this dream was telling me that, no matter what the odds, I needed to persevere. Its most important message to me was to never give up.

Author's Spirit-Led Interpretation: This dream is intended to discourage you and make you feel as though you cannot overcome the things that people are speaking to you or about you. God wants you to focus on the table that He has prepared for you in the midst of your enemies and know that your prayer life will carry you through.

Impact/Outcome: After thirty years, I have never forgotten this dream. It keeps me going sometimes, and I continue to press on in the things that the Lord has for me to do.

Primary Metaphor(s):

Crocodiles—people's words, with a big mouth and a long, powerful tail

Table—banquet table set in the presence of your enemies (see Psalm 23:5)

Red and white—red represents prayer in this dream, and white represents purity

Tablecloth—a covering

Unseen person—the Lord

Lesson: The enemy intended this dream to be a discouragement to you, but God intervened and turned it into a dream of encouragement. The single element of color in this dream takes place when God steps in and draws directly from the Scriptures to encourage you. Not only does the table itself directly represent the banquet table set in the presence of her enemies, but the colors of the tablecloth are also significant. While red can have numerous meanings, the Holy Spirit is emphasizing prayer in this case, and white is often reflective of purity. These interwoven colors indicate that maintaining purity in her prayer life would cause it to be a place of spiritual covering or protection and a key to maintaining peace in the midst of the enemy's attacks.

Dreams such as this can provide encouragement for a person to endure great difficulty and to persevere through tremendous trials, just as it did in this case. It is important to remember that even when things look difficult, greater is He who is in you than he who is in the world (see 1 John 4:4).

Consider how closely Psalm 23 (see the ESV text below) is tied to the message that the dreamer received from this dream. Many times, elements of dreams or numbers in dreams will point to scripture verses to which the dream is calling the dreamer's attention. The table in this dream is a metaphor taken from Psalm 23:5; however, its presence is an indication that the promises of the entire Twenty-Third Psalm are available to the dreamer.

The LORD is my shepherd; I shall not want. He makes me lie down in green pastures. He leads me beside still waters. He restores my soul. He leads me in paths of righteousness for his name's sake. Even though I walk through the valley of the shadow of death, I will fear no evil, for you are with me; your rod and your staff, they comfort me. You prepare a table before me in the presence of my enemies; you anoint my head with oil; my cup overflows. Surely goodness and mercy shall follow me all the days of my life, and I shall dwell in the house of the LORD forever.

Dream 20:
Destiny Choice

 (Use the QR code to hear the dreamer give more details about the dream and its significance. If you do not have access to a QR code reader, the Web site associated with this dream is listed in the INDEX.)

Dreamer: A woman in California

Source: God

Color: Vivid colors

Dream Category: Calling dream

Dream: I was at a street fair and walking through a large crowd. Walking toward me on the other side of the road was a man [the dreamer later learned that the man in her dream was John Paul Jackson] who looked like he had just come out of the Jesus People movement. He had on a T-shirt, jeans, and flip-flops. We looked at each other and we each recognized in our spirits that the other was a Christian, without having to say a word. My husband and I followed this man to an office that had beautiful wood bookshelves filled with books going all the way to the ceiling. My husband went to the bathroom and then came back. The man led me out the back door of the office, and as I looked to my left, I saw hundreds of booths set up with colorful draperies that looked like the fabric used in Indian saris. In front of me and a little off to the right was a round table.

The man sat down at this table with several other men. There was a menu listing activities from which I was supposed to choose and then relay my choice to the people sitting at the round table. I remember a few of the items: One said "spiritual readings," and another said "brow waxing." I was too nervous to choose the spiritual readings because it seemed so New Age to me, so I thought I would take the safest route and I chose the eyebrow waxing.

Dreamer's Understanding/Interpretation: I came to understand this dream as it unfolded. God was telling me that the Holy Spirit would use someone in my life to teach me deeper things about His ways. He was also showing me that I would soon have a business related to the beauty industry and that it would involve ministry to people trapped in the New Age movement. My understanding of the interpretation of this dream has grown over the years, as some of these things have come to pass in my life.

Author's Spirit-Led Interpretation: The Holy Spirit is guiding you into a ministry that will have an impact upon the New Age community. God will send people to help you understand this calling and to help you gain the knowledge you need to operate in it. He is calling attention to His vision for your life. The doors into this ministry will open first through safe, less "spiritual" things.

Impact/Outcome: About a week after I had this dream, a friend invited me to go to a conference where the man from my dream was speaking. I had never seen this man before, but after I found out who he was, I realized that I had read one of his books a few months before. The man in my dream was John Paul Jackson, and at the conference he spoke for a bit about dreams. My husband and I were in transition in ministry at the time, and we began looking at John Paul's website and found the Bridge. We visited a Bridge church in California, and the pastor there believed that we should go on a pastors' cruise to get to know some other leaders in the church. We went, and while on the cruise, we made the decision to move to Florida to sit under one of the Bridge pastors. During that time, my husband and I took all the Streams Ministries classes. A few years later, we moved back to California, and I started a skin-care company in the spa industry, which is very New Age in that part of the country.

Primary Metaphor(s):

"Jesus People" man (literally John Paul Jackson)—this man had a significant ministry to the New Age community, including interpreting dreams and sharing prophetic words or "spiritual readings." In this case, John Paul represents the Holy Spirit and His wisdom for this type of ministry.

Books—knowledge

Round table with people sitting at it—the opportunity for relationship and interaction with others

Eyebrow waxing—calling attention to the eyes, from which vision comes

Lesson: Understanding a dream can come in a moment or it can develop over a period of time. Calling dreams, such as this one, often provide an incentive to pursue something, but they don't initially provide all of the details concerning the path to get there. Dreams can also have layers of meaning that peel back with the passage of time. If at first a dream is not fully understood or does not make sense, have patience and allow the Holy Spirit to open it up to you in His timing.

This dream also provides an illustration of how God can use people as symbols. In this case, John Paul Jackson is present for two reasons. In waking life, the dreamer would eventually meet John Paul and receive training in dream interpretation and revelation ministry from him. In addition, the function or role that John Paul Jackson played in the dreamer's life was also a metaphor for the type of training and equipping that the Holy Spirit wanted to provide.

The reader board from which the dreamer had to choose services is also an interesting metaphor. One "choice" spoke to the spiritual/revelatory calling that the dreamer had, but was not yet ready to walk into fully, while the other spoke of the natural/business activities that would eventually open the doors for the dreamer and her husband to enter into their calling. However, the latter—eyebrow waxing—is not limited to a single metaphorical meaning. On the one hand, it relates to the business activity, but it also has a deeper level of meaning. Eyes are frequently a metaphor for vision or revelation, which was the area of ministry to which the dreamer was being called. Waxing the eyebrows is done to accentuate the beauty of the face, and in particular to call attention to the eyes. So, at this level, the metaphor is related to the process through which God would take the dreamer in order for her to see more clearly and care for the vision and revelation that He would be providing.

Dream 21:
Direction

Dreamer: A man in Ohio

Source: God

Color: Vivid colors

Dream Category: Direction dream

Dream: In my dream, I was raised up above the United States. Each state was a different color and had a black border around it, with a dark hue of the color also along each border. When I looked, I saw a flood moving out through the United States and into Canada, like fingers on a hand. Looking down on the map, I found myself hovering over South Carolina, and I saw what I thought was a river of dirty water. As the water flowed out, it became more and more clear. Then I began to see miracles taking place: A dead man rose up and walked; a lame man walked without his cane; a man who had no eye socket had one instantly appear; and a man with a missing arm grew a new one. I saw four worship services in churches filled to capacity, and then I felt the light mist of rain coming down for a short period of time. The air around me became a reddish-orange, like sunshine shining through a gem. I seemed to be at the end of a rainbow. I heard thunder in the east, and I was puzzled because the rain had just stopped falling.

Dreamer's Understanding/Interpretation: I knew that this dream gave me instructions on where and what I was supposed to do.

Author's Spirit-Led Interpretation: There is something significant that the Lord has for you to do in South Carolina. God wants you to see and engage in a move that will have a far-reaching impact. There is a treasure waiting to be discovered and then given away.

Impact/Outcome: After receiving further confirmation, the dreamer moved from Ohio to South Carolina to be in position for what God wanted him to do and to see. Shortly after moving to South Carolina, the dreamer had the opportunity to pray for an individual who was on life support with a pancreatic infection. The next morning, life support was removed, and the man was released from the hospital shortly thereafter. Sometime later, the dreamer prayed for a man near his home who was walking around with a cane; she saw him healed to the point of no longer needing to use the cane.

Primary Metaphor(s):

Map and positioning over South Carolina—the indication that something significant is upcoming for the dreamer in South Carolina

River—a cleansing move of the Spirit

End of the rainbow—a place where the treasure is located

Lesson: The rainbow ending in South Carolina in this dream seems to indicate that there is a significance to the geographic location; however, as in this case, most direction dreams need additional confirmation before a person should simply pack up and move to a new location. While a dream can certainly provide clear direction to take a specific action, it is always wise to be certain that you have heard God clearly. How much revelation is necessary before a person should take action on God's instruction? This is a difficult question to answer, because it is never good to wait too long, nor is it good to move too quickly. If God speaks audibly from heaven or if you encounter God in His throne room, this clearly requires little or no additional confirmation. On the other hand, simply having a feeling or experiencing a dream may necessitate additional confirmation from the Lord before a major decision is acted upon.

With something special waiting in South Carolina, when the further confirmation came, the dreamer was able to see his need to make a physical move and respond accordingly. Being a part of the prayer process that resulted in miracles that were foretold in the dream brought the dreamer the assurance he needed that he had understood the dream correctly and that he was indeed following God by making the sacrifice to move across the country and operate in his God-given calling.

Dream 22: Awakening

Dreamer: Same dreamer as *Dream 21: Direction*

Source: God

Color: Vivid colors

Dream Category: Calling dream

Dream: I was riding a motorcycle on an interstate, and I was keeping up with traffic. Then the traffic began to slow down and finally stopped. While I was sitting there talking to others who had their windows rolled down, we heard that there had been a bad wreck ahead. I managed to make it over a berm, where I could drive up to the site of the accident. I saw three medics walking back toward their vehicles shaking their heads. When they got close enough, I asked, "Is it okay if I . . ."—but before I could finish my question, I heard a voice over my right shoulder saying, "Go and pray for them." When I turned to look in the direction of the voice, I saw a man who looked familiar, but I could not place who he was. I asked the medics who the injured man was, and they told me he was "Dave." When we arrived at the scene where the mangled body was lying, the unknown man and I both knelt down beside him. Just as I was going to speak, the other man declared with great authority, "David, in the name of Jesus, rise up and be healed!" He sat right up, and after we witnessed the Gospel to him, he accepted the Lord as his Savior. We told him to sit there and we would send the medics back to him. As we reached the medics, I told them that Dave had just woken up, and without hesitation they headed back to tend to him. When I got back to my motorcycle, I saw that the other man had been riding a motorcycle, as well. The emergency personnel moved their vehicles, and we rode side by side down the road. Both motorcycles were white.

Dreamer's Understanding/Interpretation: I knew that someone was waiting on me and that I needed to go out into the world like the disciples did.

Author's Spirit-Led Interpretation: You have a calling to minister healing to others, but you have been in a place where that purpose has been hindered. The Lord wants to awaken it in you and help you to realize your full potential as His beloved child. Step out and make a move to go with Him where He is leading you.

Impact/Outcome: Because of the interpretation that indicated the need to go with the Lord, the dream provided the confirmation of a previous dream, and the dreamer subsequently moved to South Carolina, where he began to be more fully involved in ministry to others and praying for their healing.

Primary Metaphor(s):

Dave/David—this name means "cherished, beloved"

Motorcycle—a small but mobile purpose or ministry

Unknown man—the Lord

Lesson: Although the primary interpretation of this dream was about a restoration of the calling and a fulfillment of that purpose in the dreamer's life, this dream also confirmed in the heart of the dreamer that the instruction to make a geographical move, as revealed in a previous dream, was correct. In this case, the dreamer was himself in the dream, but his gifting was represented by Dave, whose motorcycle had wrecked. Remember that dreams do not have to follow the logical rules of reality. A person's life can be represented by being in the dream themselves, by being represented by another symbol in the dream (remember that Nebuchadnezzar was symbolized as a tree and a trunk in the dream that Daniel interpreted for him), or be represented by both.

The meaning of names can carry great significance in a dream. In this case, the name Dave/David means "beloved" or "cherished." The dreamer was cherished by God, but his ministry/purpose had been damaged or wounded by circumstances that had occurred along his journey in life. His purpose had been cut short, as evidenced by the medics calling him "Dave" (a shortened form of "David"), but God wanted to bring about the restoration of his full purpose, as the Lord called him "David"—the complete form of the name. God loved the gifts He had given to the dreamer and He wanted to see the dreamer use them to their fullest potential. The dream was a call to an awakening and the restoration of the dreamer's purpose and destiny that would put his natural life back on a parallel course with his spiritual calling.

Dream 23: Computer Spider

(Use the QR code to hear the dreamer give more details about the dream and its significance. If you do not have access to a QR code reader, the Web site associated with this dream is listed in the INDEX.)

Dreamer: A mother in Alabama

Source: The enemy

Color: Normal/muted colors

Dream Category: Warning dream

Dream: I was trying to chase down and catch a spider-like thing that was made up of computer parts. Its behavior was very erratic, and it was hard to catch. We kept it cornered for a while, justifying that its freedom would allow us to learn from it. Eventually I did capture it, but it kept trying to get out of the box in which I had placed it.

Dreamer's Understanding/Interpretation: A friend helped me to understand that this dream related to a computer game that was consuming my son's life.

Author's Spirit-Led Interpretation: This dream is about an attack that is coming against your family through the computer. It may not be easy to "catch" on to how this is happening, but once you do, you will be able to see that it must be dealt with or it will keep coming back.

Impact/Outcome: We didn't get rid of the computer game immediately, even though it had some occult properties to it. Instead we tried to corral it by restricting how long my son could play it and what he could do within the game. But these restrictions didn't really help. Our son just became frustrated because he couldn't play the game the way he wanted to and because he didn't like the fact that we had planned to eventually get rid of the game altogether.

Primary Metaphor(s):

Spider made of computer parts—computer-based demonic influence

Kept trying to get it out—the issue will keep coming back until it is dealt with

Lesson: The primary metaphor in this dream is an unnatural creature that is a combination of two distinct images. The first symbol is the spider, but the second was comprised of the computer parts. Remembering that dreams do not always follow natural explanations, it is important to ask, "Why was a spider made up of computer parts, instead of being a normal spider?" The why-this-and-not-that type of question can provide an opportunity to hear the voice of the Holy Spirit in a fresh, new way. In this case, the spider represents a demonic attack—something that traps its prey in a web and sucks the life out of it. Computer parts in this case have a quite natural meaning, even though the "computer spider" is far from normal. When looking at the "why" of this image, it becomes apparent that the computer parts identify the type of demonic attack that the enemy is seeking to use.

This dream and the next one, which is related to it, indicate that God is willing to keep speaking to us until we hear what He is saying. However, our response to what He is saying determines the outcome of the situation. Even when dreams are interpreted and the message is clear, how we apply or respond to the message is essential. While we often want God to loudly shout and tell us what we need to do in our times of greatest need, He is often whispering so that we draw near to Him in order to hear and understand His message to us.

There are four basic aspects to understanding a dream and what to do with it. First comes the revelation itself—the experience of God speaking to His people. Second is the interpretation—the understanding of what it is that God is trying to tell His people. Third is the application—gaining insight into how the Lord wants His people to respond to what He is saying. And finally comes the proclamation—deciding whether this is something that should be shared with others. This dream helps us to understand how important the application is to get all that God wants us to receive from a dream. If we hear the Lord and recognize what He is saying, but then we do not act on what He has revealed, we will not gain the full benefit that He intended for us, no matter how much we may talk about it or tell others how important it is.

Dream 24:
Herobrine in the Basement

 (Use the QR code to hear the dreamer give more details about the dream and its significance. If you do not have access to a QR code reader, the Web site associated with this dream is listed in the INDEX.)

Dreamer: Son of the previous dreamer in Alabama

Source: The enemy

Color: Muted colors

Dream Category: Fear dream

Dream: Herobrine, a character from a computer video game, was in the basement of my house, trying to kill me.

Dreamer's Understanding/Interpretation: The mother, having had the previous dream entitled *Computer Spider*, was immediately aware that the computer game that her son had been playing was having a negative impact upon his life.

Author's Spirit-Led Interpretation: There is something you are involved in that seems helpful, but it is actually quite destructive. This issue is affecting you at a very basic or foundational level in your life.

Impact/Outcome: The mother immediately removed the game from the house, and although it caused a great deal of frustration and anger in the dreamer, things began to improve in the home from that point forward.

Primary Metaphor(s):

Herobrine—this character's name is a play on words, or a pun. The character is not the "hero" he appears to be, but rather something that will make you sick.

Basement—something below the surface or at a foundational level

Trying to kill the dreamer—this does not necessarily indicate physical death, but it almost certainly implies an attempt to kill the dreamer's spiritual life

Lesson: The wordplay or pun alone (Hero/Brine) is almost sufficient to provide a complete interpretation. Something that appears to be a hero or beneficial is actually more "brine" in its nature. *Brine* is water saturated strongly with salt. What looks like it could be used to quench a person's thirst, if consumed, is more likely to make one sick. In other words, a villain is masquerading as a hero in the dreamer's life.

It may seem strange that the Lord would use such a pun to convey such a serious message; however, it is important to remember that God will speak in whatever fashion that will make His message clear. The enemy is not a creator, but rather a counterfeiter. In this case, his failure was in the lack of creativity in the choice of a name for the hero of the computer video game. While this may seem humorous at first glance, it is important to recognize that a "merry heart is good like a medicine" (see Proverbs 17:22), and in this case, it refers to a "medicine" that the dreamer did not even realize he was taking.

Additionally, this dream illustrates how the Lord can allow a dream from the enemy to be used for His purposes. The mother dream had not yet fully responded to her own dream, but her son's dream from the enemy helped her to see the impact that the computer video game was having on her son, and she began to more fully respond to the instruction she had received in her own dream.

Dream 25:
Yeshua: A God Who Saves

Dreamer: A mother in Auckland, New Zealand

Source: The enemy

Color: Muted colors

Dream Category: Fear dream

Dream: I dreamed that I was walking through sand dunes with my husband, my father, and my children. The children ran on ahead, but the area was vast, and we could clearly see them ahead of us, so we were not too worried. Then the ground began to shake, and the sand started moving. I saw my daughter disappear down into the sand. I screamed and ran to the place where I thought I'd seen her last and began frantically digging in the sand. My father was digging beside me. We could not get to her in time, but we found her outstretched hand reaching up.

Dreamer's Understanding/Interpretation: The dreamer did not receive an interpretation, nor did she understand the dream until it came to pass.

Author's Spirit-Led Interpretation: This dream is calling you to prayer for your children. God, your Father, is with you always and can clearly see what lies before you. Though the things of the world may seek to envelop you or your loved ones, He is always there to help you. Do not allow the enemy to cause you to fear or to fall into a place of despair.

Impact/Outcome: I agonized over this dream for months. Every time I thought of my little girl's hand reaching up for me, I broke down in tears. During the summer holidays, we spent time at my parents' house, where there is a big swimming pool that our children love. One day my husband was playing on the steps with our six-month-old son, and I was on the other side of the fence talking about what we would do that afternoon. Out of the blue, I had a horrible panicky feeling, like I had had in the dream, and I looked over to where our other children were swimming. I couldn't see my daughter anywhere. Then I caught sight of her hand stretched up out of the water—in exactly the same position as it had been stretched up out of the sand in my dream. I cried out, and my husband pulled her up out of the water. Although she was shaken and upset, she was okay. Without a doubt, God had alerted us to the situation and saved her life that day, and I realized He was right beside me, just as He had been in my dream.

Primary Metaphor(s):

Sand dunes—the earth, or the things of the earth

Father—God, the heavenly Father

"We could not get to her in time, but we found her outstretched hand reaching up"—a lie that God is not sufficient to preserve the dreamer's family. This is the element of fear that the enemy was seeking to project.

Lesson: It is important to recognize that even dreams from the enemy can provide hope, when a Spirit-led interpretation is provided. Here, the dream was intended to create fear in the dreamer, but it also gave away a specific type of attack that the enemy was planning and it allowed the dreamer to prepare for that attack, although in this case, the preparation was not conscious or intentional.

Even when a dream is not fully understood by our natural minds, it does not mean that our spirits fail to comprehend it. A lack of natural understanding allowed the enemy to provoke ongoing fear in the dreamer, but her inner consciousness regarding the dream's purpose kept the potential attack in the foreground and resulted in ongoing prayer. Keep in mind that these outcomes could have been brought to pass without the anxiety that came from the failure to understand the dream, had there been a Spirit-led interpretation available before the dream actually came to pass.

The enemy attempts to instill fear through dreams for a number of reasons. While general nightmares are often designed to cause the dreamer to reject dreams as a means of hearing God's voice, specific anxiety-producing dreams, such as this one, frequently reveal some element of the enemy's plan of attack. In such cases, it is helpful to "flip the dream." While this does not simply mean to look for the dream's opposite meaning, it does allow us to apply the principle that what the enemy intends for evil, God will use for good (see Genesis 50:20). In this case, the message of fear the enemy intended to implant through the dream was that God's oversight was insufficient to protect the family, but God used that very dream, which the enemy had intended for the installation of fear, to provide a warning and the assurance that He would preserve the life of the dreamer's precious child.

Dream 26:
Don't Listen to the Cobra

Dreamer: A man in Alabama

Source: God

Color: Normal colors

Dream Category: Intercessory dream

Dream: In my dream, I was observing my mother as she sat in a chair in her living room. Near her chair was a potter's wheel spinning, and on the wheel was a large cobra that was standing on its tail and took the shape of a large S. As I watched, my mother reached out, took the snake at the base of its head, and touched its mouth to her ear, so that its tongue could flick in and out. My mother then tried to hand the snake to my wife, but she refused to take it.

Dreamer's Understanding/Interpretation: I knew when I woke up that this dream was calling me to pray for my mother and that the enemy was trying influence her thoughts.

Author's Spirit-Led Interpretation: This dream is a call to prayer. Your mother is allowing the enemy to "tickle her ear" with his lies, and he wants her to pass on this deception to the next generation.

Impact/Outcome: I had been asking the Lord for direction on how to pray for my mother, and this dream was a direct answer. I was concerned about whether my mother was suffering solely from a physical or mental condition, or whether part of the issue was related to a spiritual attack against her. After experiencing this dream, I was better equipped to pray and to respond to her with a greater level of understanding.

Primary Metaphor(s):

Mother—in this case, the mother is not a metaphor but the dreamer's literal mother

Potter's wheel—a place where something takes shape or is formed

Wife—the mother of the next generation

Cobra—a high level of demonic lies and deceit

Lesson: Notice that the dreamer does not appear anywhere in this dream. Dreams in which the dreamer is observing others and is not present in the dream can be considered extrinsic in nature—that is, they are about something other than the dreamer themselves. Extrinsic dreams are not extremely common, because most dreams are about the dreamer's life rather than about others. In most cases, extrinsic dreams are either prophetic or intercessory in nature. Because extrinsic dreams provide revelation or call the dreamer to prayer about a third party or an outside circumstance, it is far more common (although not exclusive) for spiritual leaders, prophetic intercessors, and prayer warriors to have this type of dream.

This particular dream gives the dreamer insight as to how to pray for his mother. While the mother was battling various physical, mental, and emotional issues, the Lord wanted the dreamer to recognize that this was ultimately a spiritual conflict and it needed to be properly addressed in prayer. The potter's wheel indicates that this attack is still in the process of taking shape and it is not fully developed. It provides encouragement to the dreamer that spiritual warfare could change the outcome.

Dream Stories by Michael B. French

Dream 27:
A Walk in the River

Dreamer: A woman in Alabama

Source: God

Color: Black and white, but turning into normal colors

Dream Category: Healing dream

Dream: In my dream, it was very dark, and I was in a wide creek with many stones. The water was very nasty and thick. I was also very nasty. I was crawling because I couldn't walk. My dress was dirty, and I smelled bad. On the bank of the creek, I could see all the people who had hurt me. They were all looking down on me, because I was so dirty and helpless. This is what they had been telling me for years. This went on for some time, and then I began to see a light in the distance. The water started to clear up, and I got more and more clean the closer I moved toward the light. I was finally able to stand as the water continued cleaning me. My dress became white, and my shoulder-length hair became clean. I realized that I was barefooted, and all the people who had been on the bank were now gone. New people were there now, dressed in white clothes, and I realized that the light was Jesus Himself. I reached out to Him, and I was safe.

Dreamer's Understanding/Interpretation: I understood this dream to mean that the world was the dark place of filth and the rocks were troubles and hardheartedness, but that the closer I got to Jesus, the cleaner I would become.

Author's Spirit-Led Interpretation: Your life has been filled with trials, and there have been many people around you who have hurt you and spoken ill of you, but God has a purpose for you. As you trust Him more and more, He will wash away the hurt and pain, bringing His value to your life.

Impact/Outcome: I have never forgotten this dream, though I had it many years before. It helped me realize that staying close to God would keep me from being overcome by all the hurt and darkness that I had experienced.

Primary Metaphor(s):

Stones—trials, challenges, and stumbling blocks

Critical people looking down—those who had spoken ill of the dreamer

White clothes—transformation

Bare feet—peace

Lesson: Dreams such as this help to bring an awareness that it is not how others see us, but rather how we are seen by ourselves and by our Creator that is most important. Healing dreams often help the dreamers to recognize and overcome things that they would not be able to consciously process and relinquish. In this case, by pressing past what others had said and drawing closer to Jesus, the dreamer was able to find strength to forgive and overcome all that had been difficult in her waking life. She could then take that spiritual strength and apply it to her day-to-day reality.

The transformation took place in the dream first, causing faith to arise in the dreamer that what had happened in the dream could also manifest in waking life. While the dreamer might have known the hurt that others had caused in her life, this dream brought that pain to a focal point that she could see and feel, as opposed to a collection of feelings that spanned the dreamer's lifetime, and the dream demonstrated that the enemy had tried to separate the issues and convince her that their individual impact was not worth dealing with. Seeing the pain that had been caused collectively allowed the dreamer to recognize the freedom that the Lord desired to bring and to trust the transformation that God was working in her life.

Being barefoot might seem to convey the idea of vulnerability, but the path had been sufficiently smoothed to allow it to be walked across safely. Notice how many different images convey the idea of transformation: the water changes from nasty to clean; the clothes change from dirty to white; the people on the bank change from accusing to encouraging; the progress changes from crawling to walking; and the atmosphere changes from dark to light. All of these images speak to the importance that God places on seeing the dreamer walking in healing and wholeness.

Dream 28:
Slow Down So You Don't Get Hurt

Dreamer: A mother in Alabama

Source: God

Color: Normal colors

Dream Category: Intercessory dream

Dream: I was watching my son drive a car on a narrow, elevated road in a big city. He was coming around a curve. Cars were parked on the shoulder, making it difficult to drive down the narrow road. My son came through in his car and was bumping the other vehicles as he passed. I was worried about him bumping these cars, and I was worried that he would get hurt.

Dreamer's Understanding/Interpretation: At first, I thought the dream meant that my son might need prayer for his ministry, so that he didn't hurt himself or others, but he really wasn't in any specific kind of ministry at that time.

Author's Spirit-Led Interpretation: Pray for your son so that neither he nor those around him will be hurt as he navigates the path before him.

Impact/Outcome: Even though I misunderstood the dream, I prayed for my son anyway. While traveling to an event with some college friends a few days later, he was involved in an automobile accident in which he broke his leg. I then realized what the dream had meant. The car in which he had been riding had been hit directly in the passenger side, and his injuries should have been much more significant. I know that the prayer—prompted by the dream—protected him.

Primary Metaphor(s):

Son—literally the dreamer's son

Car—vocation, in this case a student

Narrow road—a person's journey or path

Lesson:

Vehicles are the means by which we get from one place to another. Dreams about vehicles can have to do with either a spiritual journey or a natural one. Ministry, in its broadest form, is the vehicle used to get us from one point in our spiritual journey to another, and our vocation is the vehicle used to get us from one point to another in our natural journey. This similarity indicates how important it is for the dreamer to remain dependent upon the Holy Spirit to distinguish between the possible meanings of any individual symbol. Here, the dreamer initially mistook the meaning of the car, but she allowed the Holy Spirit to draw her attention to its appropriate meaning by recognizing her difficulty in applying the dream due to her erroneous interpretation of symbol of the car.

Even though this dream was initially misinterpreted, knowing its purpose was significant. The fact that this dream was a call to prayer was not hindered whatsoever by the initial misunderstanding. By praying both in relationship to how the dream was initially understood and also generally asking God to provide His protection for her son, the dreamer was able to respond to the dream appropriately.

It is important to trust God for understanding and to recognize that even though some interpretations are unclear until the dream comes to pass, God can still direct our steps, though the message He sends may remain partially veiled. In this case, had God revealed the full understanding of the dream, it is possible that the mother would have responded in fear instead of faith, and perhaps she would have become overprotective rather than dependent upon God's protection.

Dream 29:
The Twins

Dreamer: A woman in Georgia, in June 2005

Source: God

Color: Vivid colors

Dream Category: Prophetic/Intercessory dream

Dream: I was standing on a beautiful, sunny beach. I could see a storm coming in from the distant sky and many small hurricanes all beside one another being formed in the ocean. I was yelling for my nephew named Brent, who lives in Florida, to come inside, but I couldn't find him anywhere. I could see people running in to get off the beach, and when I looked into the distance again, I could see two massive hurricanes coming forward quickly. They were side by side, and giant words had formed between them that read "The Twins."

Dreamer's Understanding/Interpretation: There was a strong sense of urgency in this dream, and I understood it to mean that two hurricanes were about to hit the United States.

Author's Spirit-Led Interpretation: Like a watchman on a hill, you are being called to pray for protection from the storms (whether literal or spiritual) that are coming.

Impact/Outcome: In August and September, Hurricanes Katrina and Rita hit the United States' Gulf Coast. Much like twins, these storms had many similarities in appearance, but each acted and were responded to quite differently.

Primary Metaphor(s):

Hurricanes—storms or trials, but in this case, they were literal

Brent—the name means "hilltop"

Yelling for nephew—a call to prayer and/or a warning

Lesson: There can be a tendency to assume that a prophetic dream requires a public announcement of its revelation. While this can certainly be significant in certain situations, prayer should always be the first response to such a dream. In this particular dream, the symbols themselves tend to point the dreamer to prayer rather than proclamation. A watchman may be set upon a hilltop, but it can also be a high place or a place from which prayers can be raised. The call of the dreamer was not necessarily for everyone to evacuate the coast, but for her to come up to the hilltop and lift her voice in prayer.

It is not always clear when a prophetic dream is actually a prophetic dream; however, it is always appropriate to pray based upon what the dream reveals. The nature of a prophetic dream does not mandate that the dreamer deliver a message to everyone, but it always calls the dreamer to intercession.

Once the first hurricane began to develop, it would have become much clearer to the dreamer that the dream was more directly prophetic, and by the time the second hurricane in the Gulf had emerged, the dreamer would have certainly been more comfortable calling others to prayer. In this case, both the natural development of Rita and the response of people were improvements over that of Katrina, and such changes can be at least partially attributed to increased prayer raised by dreams such as this one and other prophetic warnings.

Dream 30:
Escaping the Spider

Dreamer: A woman in Alabama

Source: God

Color: Normal colors with gray-scale elements

Dream Category: Self-condition dream

Dream: In my dream, I was sleeping in my apartment. A noise woke me up. When I opened my eyes, my room, closet, hallway, and bathroom all had a *huge* spiderweb woven through them. I sat up screaming. When I sat up, I could feel the stickiness of the web. The dream was in color, but the web was not; it was dark gray. The web was strong, too. I couldn't move, because the spider had woven its web all around me. I started screaming, because I realized that I was trapped. Apparently, when I screamed, the spider realized that I had awakened. I could hear it coming down the hallway, attempting to weave more of its web while it came back toward me. I started screaming again, because I knew that if I did not get out of my apartment filled with the huge spiderweb, the spider would eat me alive. Then I woke up.

Dreamer's Understanding/Interpretation: No one interpreted this dream for me, but over the years since, I have come to understand that it related to the occult activity in my life and how I had been bound by its effects on me. I know that God was awakening my spirit to accept Him and be set free.

Author's Spirit-Led Interpretation: This dream is revealing the condition of your life. You are bound up in something dark that is going to consume you if you don't receive the help you need to get free.

Impact/Outcome: The dreamer was involved in occult activity and had this dream a week before meeting a pastor who helped her to leave the occult behind, turn her life over to the Lord, and receive her freedom from the demonic strings that had bound her. The dreamer said that she would not have listened to the pastor, nor believed that she was bound by her occult activities, had it not been for this dream.

Primary Metaphor(s):

Spider—occult attack or activity

Web—the trap created by occult activity

Gray—compromise, lifelessness

Apartment—life; the place where you are living temporarily

Lesson: Webs are sticky and tend to hold things in place. In this dream, the dreamer felt trapped by the things going on in her life at the time of the dream. The gray color of the web might be considered a "natural" color, but the emphasis that the dreamer felt on the "dark gray" nature of the web helps identify that it also has significance for the dream's meaning. Gray is a color that is neither black nor white, thus representing compromise, or in this case, a place in the dreamer's life where she had not made wise choices and where the enemy was trapping her in order to drain her life.

This dream revealed to the dreamer the condition that her life was in and the danger that it involved. The color in the dream helps identify this dream as being from God, but the gray web revealed the enemy's plan to destroy the dreamer. This dream is an excellent example of how God can allow the enemy to insert elements into dreams that He gives, so that a person can more clearly see the enemy's plan. Black-and-white or muted-color dreams from the enemy can also have color elements inserted into them that demonstrate how God is able to overcome the darkness (see John 1:5).

Dream 31:
Little Blind Girl

(Use the QR code to hear the dreamer give more details about the dream and its significance. If you do not have access to a QR code reader, the Web site associated with this dream is listed in the INDEX.)

Dreamer: A woman in West Virginia

Source: God

Color: Color

Dream Category: Self-condition dream

Dream: I dreamed of a young girl about whom I was concerned. I feel like I was trying to take care of her or hide and shelter her, because she was very vulnerable. It seemed that whoever had created her had abandoned her. My husband and I were in a line with her, and people were passing through that line greeting us. The child (although she thought she was a woman) seemed to be drawn to particular men in the line. Then I realized that she was blind and she was not aware that she was being drawn to certain men. These men looked like foreign dignitaries or members of the nobility. They were dressed very formally and they looked to be very influential. I told one of the men in the line to speak to her in his native tongue to see her reaction, because I knew she was Asian. He spoke to her, and I could tell that she recognized the connection. It seemed as if she had been created blind so that she would not make this connection. I remember seeing a woman sitting cross-legged in a costume-type dress in the dusty street of a market area, and I thought that she was the one who had created this child. I did not feel good about this person. She was responsible for the child's being blind. I remember thinking that the child was so beautiful, but she was blind. I was sad that she did not know that she was Asian, and that the truth had been hidden from her.

Dreamer's Understanding/Interpretation: The little girl is me. The culture in which I was raised had prevented me from seeing spiritually who God had created me to be. I am a child of the King, and therefore I am royalty. I have an inheritance from God that He wants me to understand and receive. This dream was the beginning of my journey to receiving that inheritance.

Author's Spirit-Led Interpretation: This dream is about you. The spiritual environment around you has blinded you to the understanding of who you are and the purpose for which you were created. God is showing you that you are an important part of the Kingdom and that you relate to and can communicate with the King.

Impact/Outcome: I did not understand that the little girl was me for quite a while. I kept thinking about the dream, and God gradually showed me that the girl was me. This was the second dream that I recorded in my dream journal, and so it was a very significant dream that started my journey into finding out who I really am in Christ Jesus. I am no longer blind, and now my passion is to teach others how to spiritually begin to "see" and find their place in God's Kingdom.

Primary Metaphor(s):

Little girl—the dreamer

Blindness—the inability to perceive

Dignitaries and nobility—representatives of the Kingdom of God

Cross-legged woman—a religious spirit

Lesson: Blindness represents the inability to see or to perceive something, and in this dream, it is the inability to see the connection with the nobility that represents the Kingdom of God. Here, the dreamer felt that the cross-legged woman had created this child blind, and thus had prevented her connection. The position of the woman is related to the pseudo-spirituality of gurus and shamans and thus an indication of the religious spirit, probably arising out of the church culture in which the dreamer had been raised. The Church is described in the Scriptures as the Bride of Christ, which is all about relationship. A corruption of this image would be portrayed by this woman and her pseudo-spirituality that focuses on religion and its rules rather than the intimacy born out of relationship with the King.

Typically, in order for a dream to be about the dreamer, the dreamer must be the focus of the dream or the center of attention. In this case, however, it is the little girl who is the center of attention, but the dream is still about the dreamer. This is because the dreamer is observing herself as the little girl in the dream. This is similar to Nebuchadnezzar's dream of the tree recorded in Daniel 4. The tree, not the king, was the focus of the dream, but the tree was a metaphor for the dreamer/king. Thus, in both examples, the dreams are about the dreamer, even though they are not the central focus of the dream on a surface level.

Dream 32:
Get that Mole Checked

 *(Use the QR code to hear the dreamer give more details about the dream and its significance. If you do not have access to a QR code reader, the Web site associated with this dream is listed in the INDEX.)*

Dreamer: A man in West Virginia

Source: God

Color: Normal colors

Dream Category: Warning dream

Dream: I am lying on a bed with my wife, and my head is in her lap. I feel that someone is about to come into the room, and I begin to cover her up. A lady comes into the room and points to my wife's inner left thigh. I believe she questions me and asks, "What is this?" The lady is pointing to an area on my wife's inner thigh that has a scar where a mole had been removed in the past. I see the area and it is almost the size of a dime, and the color of the area is darker in color compared to the other skin on her leg.

Dreamer's Understanding/Interpretation: The dreamer could not interpret this dream, but in waking life, his spouse took the dream to be literal.

Author's Spirit-Led Interpretation: This dream is a warning that something is out of order beneath the surface and needs to be dealt with.

Impact/Outcome: My wife made an appointment with a dermatologist to investigate a mole in the spot where the lady in the dream had indicated she should check. The diagnosis was malignant melanoma. The mole was removed, and no further treatment was needed. We had found the mole early enough to spare my wife's life.

Primary Metaphor(s):

Wife—literal

Nameless person (woman)—in this case, an angel or a messenger from God

Color (darker area)—something is out of order or doesn't fit with the rest of the image

Lesson: It can be argued that this was not a dream at all, but a vision. Many believe that a dream is something that takes place at night, while a vision is something that occurs when a person is awake. However, it is clear from the Scriptures that visions can occur during the night and they may involve encounters with spiritual beings, as well (see Daniel 4:13). As has been previously indicated, it may be more accurate to define the difference as a dream being something that is more metaphorical and a vision being something that is more literal. In this case, there is less need for interpretation as the message is more literal, thus defining this experience as fitting into the realm of a vision or perhaps a vision within a dream.

Consider the importance of the revelation provided in this dream/vision. This is literally a lifesaving warning. Had the dreamer or his spouse simply assumed that this was a dream that they did not understand and had done nothing, the consequences could have been catastrophic. Much of this dream had a very literal application and lent itself to being taken literally. In addition, there were very few negative consequences to taking it literally and having the mole checked out.

Dream 33:
My Advocate

Dreamer: A woman in Florida

Source: God

Color: Color

Dream Category: Courage dream

Dream: I walked in the front door of my attorney's office. As I waited for him, I walked out to what seemed like a back porch. There was a large banquet table with so much food on the table. I saw a white wedding cake, and I knew I would love a slice of it. Then I looked out at the yard, where the grass was very green and well cared for. I noticed there were several rows of lettuce growing across the yard. I knew one row belonged to me, but I didn't understand why.

Dreamer's Understanding/Interpretation: I was going through a difficult time and I had been worried about it, but the Lord, my advocate, was with me. He had prepared a table before me in the presence of my enemies, and the portion or provision I was to receive had already been decided. This dream was meant to encourage me.

Author's Spirit-Led Interpretation: You are in need of counsel and someone to stand with you through a trial. God has prepared a place of peace and rest for you during this difficult time, and He will keep His covenant of provision with you.

Impact/Outcome: In real life, I was dealing with a situation that involved a very good trial attorney. I was walking in fear that the attorney would prevail in the situation. I have never forgotten this dream, as it gave me peace that my Advocate would help me walk victoriously in this or in any other situation. This dream brought comfort and helped Psalm 23 become real in my life.

Primary Metaphor(s):

Attorney—an advocate, in this case an Advocate with the Father, Christ Jesus

Banquet table—a place of nourishment and a Psalm 23 place of peace

Well-cared-for green grass—a place of rest

Lettuce—money

Lesson: The lettuce in this dream could have had a number of meanings, but in this case, it was a wordplay or a pun based upon a slang use of the word *lettuce*, meant to refer to money. It is important to remember that a symbol can have multiple meanings, and both the context of the dream and the background of the dreamer can have an impact upon which meaning is appropriate to a particular dream. In order to provide a spiritual interpretation to a dream, it is essential that the interpreter be open to hear the Holy Spirit's voice as He gives insight into which symbols are important in a dream and which meanings of a symbol are correct in a particular situation.

In this case, the dreamer learned, long after interpreting the dream for herself, that the term *lettuce* could be used to refer to money. She knew that the dream was promising peace and comfort in a difficult situation, but God had hidden the meaning of the lettuce so that she would not focus on financial provision, but rather trust Him for full provision and protection in a difficult time. In cases such as this, the understanding of the symbol after the fact can easily be dismissed as no longer significant, but it is important to remember that the confirmation it provides that the dreamer was hearing clearly can be equally important.

While courage dreams such as this one can instill the courage necessary to overcome adversity or to make it through a particularly difficult season, they can also encourage dreamers that they are indeed hearing from the Lord and that He cares both about them and their circumstances.

Dream 34:
Highs and Lows of Learning Spiritual Gifts

Dreamer: A woman in Kentucky

Source: God

Color: Color

Dream Category: Calling dream

Dream: I was standing in a green, grassy area outside my house, looking up at an exceptionally blue sky, a perfect-weather day. Someone in white came up beside me (but I didn't see his face), and we began to fly. My gown was long and white. At first it was wonderful and fun, but then we started moving very high and far away from home. I became nervous and began to question the process. I looked down and saw that we were flying over an ocean. No longer able to see land, I said, "I can't fly, and I especially don't like flying over water." At that, I began a long descent, plunging into the ocean and dropping straight to the bottom. As I sat on the bottom of the ocean floor, I thought I was going to die. I held my breath for as long as I could, and I was ready to take in water, but as I gasped, I realized that I could breathe underwater. It was a little more difficult than breathing the air outside, but it was doable. I felt like a fish and wondered whether I had gills. I went sightseeing in the deep and swimming underwater until I awoke.

Dreamer's Understanding/Interpretation: I was at a time in my life when I was learning how to go higher in spiritual understanding and the capabilities the Lord had for me. It was far away from the traditional church beliefs I had had. I questioned the supernatural and my ability to operate in it. Faith in God was a key. As I begin to speak my doubt, I fell (it reminds me of Peter's walking on water and then sinking when he looked at the circumstances surrounding him). The great thing is, no matter where I found myself, God made a way, provided wonderfully, and was always with me. He wouldn't let me drown in the process, and instead, I experienced the heights and depths of His love in this dream.

Author's Spirit-Led Interpretation: God is calling you to move into a new level of your spiritual walk. It may be scary, but the journey is worth it. Even when you think you can't make it and question your own capabilities, He will take you deeper and teach you things you didn't know you could do as you live a supernatural spiritual life. The journey you are on may involve tests and challenges, but you are well-suited for it and you will become who God has created you to be.

Impact/Outcome: I was coming from a very conservative Christian background that made accepting supernatural/spiritual things difficult. This dream helped me to let go of some of my fears about how God operates and learn how to go higher spiritually. My spiritual walk has stretched me at times, but God has always taught me what I needed to know and He has never abandoned me.

Primary Metaphor(s):

Flying—moving higher into spiritual things, often a symbol of a prophetic gifting

Faceless person—the Holy Spirit

Bottom of the ocean—deep things of the Spirit

Lesson: This is one of those dreams that can seem to fit into more than one category. Some would consider this a courage dream, because it provided support for the dreamer to move forward in the things of the Spirit, but it could also fit into the calling category, as it lets the dreamer know that there is a purpose in her life, and that is where she is at the moment.

Another important lesson from this dream is to recognize that just because fear or doubt is present in a dream, that does not mean that the dream is from the enemy. Notice that in this dream, the fear, as the dreamer indicates, causes a Peter-like plunge, but she is never abandoned by the Holy Spirit. The fear and doubt present in this dream are not focused upon, but rather they are a reminder that they can be overcome, even when we don't know how to do it ourselves. It is equally important to note that in her dream, the dreamer did not want to fly, especially over water, but the rejection of her calling in the dream did not stop the fulfillment of it in her waking life. Instead, the dream simply adjusted the metaphor to allow the dreamer to recognize that whether it was viewed as the depths of the ocean or the heights of the atmosphere, the call of God on her life was inescapable.

The emotions in this dream, both those directly identified and those implied, are as powerful as the visual images the dream contains. Fun, wonder, nervousness, anxiety, fear, and excitement all play a vital role in understanding the journey on which the dreamer is traveling. The progression of these emotions seems to mirror the progression of the journey described in the dreamer's understanding of her dream. In fact, the dreamer's interpretation could almost entirely be drawn out of these emotions alone, even without an understanding of the visual images and what they represent.

Dream 35:
Mickey Mouse and Santa

Dreamer: A street gang leader in Alabama

Source: The enemy

Color: None

Dream Category: False dream

Dream: I dreamed I saw Mickey Mouse and Santa Claus beating up the Baby Jesus with a baseball bat.

Dreamer's Understanding/Interpretation: None

Author's Spirit-Led Interpretation: "Does anyone have a real dream they would like to have interpreted?"

Impact/Outcome: While interpreting dreams on the street in Birmingham, Alabama, a ministry team encountered a group of young people and asked whether any of them had had a dream they would like to have interpreted. The leader of the gang immediately volunteered, and the enemy created this lie in order to shut down any chance for this gang to receive help and support from the Lord. By the interpreter immediately declaring this dream to be false and standing up to the gang leader, other members of the gang were freed to share their dreams, including the next dream, entitled "The Blue Car."

Primary Metaphor(s):

None

Lesson: Jeremiah 23:32 speaks of God's stance against false prophets and those who use false or lying dreams. Such dreams are designed to lead people astray by their lies and recklessness. Dreams such as the one recounted here are not dreams at all, but rather lies masquerading as dreams and they are designed to be a trap that will ensnare the unsuspecting. There are no metaphors, and there is no interpretation to this particular "dream," because it was not sent by either God or the enemy. In a very loose sense, it originates in the soul of the dreamer as a fabrication designed for deception.

Not as much is learned from this so-called dream as is learned from the encounter with the dreamer. God sometimes hides things from us in order that we might respond to Him and not to our feelings, emotions, or circumstances. In this case, God blinded the eyes of the team to the fact that they were dealing with a street gang, until after the response to the gang leader had already been presented. Had the team realized whom they were dealing with, they might have operated more out of fear and not taken the bold stand of putting the gang leader in his place. The response that the Lord orchestrated created respect for the ministry team in the eyes of the other young men and women, and it allowed them to share very personal experiences with a liberty they would not otherwise have had.

Dream 36:
The Blue Car

Dreamer: A young female gang member in Alabama

Source: God

Color: Color

Dream Category: Correction dream

Dream: I dreamed that I was at my house when my boyfriend came over in a blue car. He came inside, and we had sex (the dreamer provided a more graphic description here that would not be appropriate in this context). The next day, he came over again and I was excited for him to come into the house, but when he got out of the car, he pulled out a gun and killed me.

Dreamer's Understanding/Interpretation: The meaning was unknown to the dreamer, until the Spirit interpretation was provided.

Author's Spirit-Led Interpretation: You have been battling depression, and it will attempt to kill you if you don't do something to break its influence in your life. The people to whom you feel close and with whom you have been hanging out are a part of the problem and not the solution. God gave you this dream to let you know that you can overcome this difficulty and walk into your destiny.

Impact/Outcome: The young lady immediately responded to the dream with shock. She explained that her mother had been telling her the same thing, and that she did not believe it. Her mother had begged her to go to a doctor and get on medication for depression, and she had actually made an appointment for her to see a doctor the following day.

Primary Metaphor(s):

Blue—depression

Sex—intimate relationship

Killed me—something is "killing" the dreamer

Lesson: When examining a dream such as this one, it is important to remember that the dreamer doesn't have to "get saved" in order for the dream to have a significant impact on their life. Paul said that he planted seed, that Apollos watered the seed, but that God was the One who brought the harvest (see 1 Corinthians 3:6). This is one of those cases in which the interpretation of the dream either planted or watered, but it still remained God's responsibility to bring about the harvest. Whether this young lady sought medical attention, pursued a deeper relationship with God, or did nothing at all is unknown. It is known, though, that God clearly wanted her to understand that there was an issue in her relationships that was bringing destruction into her life and that He was giving her the opportunity to respond, knowing that she could stand up to the peer pressure she was experiencing and initiate change in her life.

This dream also illustrates an important aspect of using dream interpretation as a means of evangelism. In recounting the dream for the purpose of this book, the dreamer's account was "sanitized" to make it more palatable to the reader. However, when interacting with unsaved people, it is important to remember that they are, in fact, unsaved and are not guided by the same moral compass as believers are, nor do they engage the same verbal filters that more mature Christians tend to use. If dream interpreters react rashly or with shock to the particular language used or the specific imagery that an unsaved person encountered in a dream, they may very well shut down an opportunity to share the message of Jesus with someone who desperately needs to hear it. While a more thorough examination of the negative impact that culture shock can have on evangelistic efforts is beyond the scope of this book, it is important to remember that God is not as easily offended as we are, and as He did in this case, He will touch the life of an individual regardless of their present situation or circumstances.

Dream 37:
My Dying Mom

Dreamer: A woman in Florida

Source: God

Color: Color

Dream Category: Calling dream

Dream: I dreamed that my mom was sitting at a dinner table and was struck by a lightning bolt. In my dream, she died immediately.

Dreamer's Understanding/Interpretation: Fear that my mother would physically die

Author's Spirit-led Interpretation: Your mother is about to be impacted by the power of God in such a way that who she was will die so that she can come alive to who she was created to be.

Impact/Outcome: Initially, this dream created fear about my mother, but when the dream was interpreted, it brought hope. The interpretation described exactly what soon occurred in my mother's life. She has totally changed and is now on fire for God.

Primary Metaphor(s):

Lightning bolt—power, in this case the power of God

Death—death to the old man

Lesson: This is a great example of how a dream that was given by God can still produce fear in our lives when it is not understood correctly. Attempting to apply a soulish interpretation to a spiritual dream will produce no fruit. On the other hand, remember that applying a spiritual interpretation to a soulish dream can still bring life from the dream. When a loved one dies in a dream from God, it is uncommon for the dream to indicate that the loved one is going to physically die (although it is not totally unheard of; in these cases, however, there are usually other elements of the dream that indicate that it is intended to prepare the dreamer for such a loss). In almost every case, the death of a loved one in a dream speaks of a spiritual transformation and dying to the old nature so that something new can come forth.

While this dream has been categorized as a calling dream, it is important to realize that most calling dreams relate to the dreamer's own life and not the life of someone else. In this case, however, the close relationship of the dreamer to the focus of the dream (a parent/child relationship) provides hope for the dreamer that God was about to move in her mother's life and that the call of God was going to be fulfilled. For these reasons, this dream could also easily be categorized as an intercessory dream.

Dream 38:
She's Alive

Dreamer: A woman in West Virginia

Source: God

Color: Color

Dream Category: Healing dream

Dream: I was in a room standing all alone, when my mother came walking through the door. Her face was radiant and glowing, and she was young again. I was so excited to see her. I said, "Mom, is that you?" She said, "It's me." I replied, "You're not dead!" She said, "I'm not dead." I then yelled for my brothers and my sisters to come. They all came and ran up to her and embraced her. Then another door opened from the back of the room, and it was *her* brothers and sisters and they all ran to her, and all of us just hugged her, and we were all so happy to see her. She was dressed in a very bright fuchsia color. I woke up and began to cry because it had seemed so real.

Dreamer's Understanding/Interpretation: My mother is not dead, but alive with the Lord, and one day I will see her again.

Author's Spirit-Led Interpretation: The Lord wants you to know that your mother is not dead, but alive (see Mark 12:27), and she is growing in a new understanding of her royal priesthood (see 1 Peter 2:9). Do not fear: You will see her again one day.

Impact/Outcome: This dream brought me comfort, as my mother had recently died from breast cancer, and I was dealing with grief. The dream helped me to recognize that my mother was much more alive with the Lord than she had been on earth, and that we would be reunited one day.

Primary Metaphor(s):

Mother—in this case literal

Family gathering—there will be a reunion

Fuchsia dress—growing royalty

Lesson: Dreams of deceased loved ones can be challenging. All too often, individuals who have lost loved ones become obsessed with asking God to "let me see them again," and thus they are focused on their own sense of how peace and comfort should come to them. A person should never be encouraged to seek out a visitation from a deceased person, as this is akin to necromancy. On the other hand, when God chooses to comfort an individual by allowing them to see a deceased loved one in a dream, there is no biblical prohibition. The primary distinction is based upon who initiates the encounter: God or man. In this case, the sense of peace and comfort brought in the dream and the dreamer's lack of desire to repeat such an encounter in her own strength helps to establish that this dream was from the Lord.

The color fuchsia is an interesting image in this dream. Fuchsia is not a common color that is described frequently in dreams, though it is a well-known color. Frequently, when describing colors, dreamers stick to the basic color palette, at times even when a more exotic description would be appropriate. Thus, specifically referencing "fuchsia" is a significant element of this dream. Fuchsia is a vivid, purplish red, but it is not the deep purple normally associated with royalty or royal robes, so in this case it represents royalty that is not yet at its fullest completion. Revelation 1:6 describes God's people as kings and priests, and because the mother in this dream had only recently died, the imagery is that of just entering her royal position in heaven.

Also, remember that healing dreams can heal a broken heart, a broken relationship, or even a broken bone. A healing dream helps enable individuals to overcome some pain or hurt that exists in their lives, whether it be physical, mental, emotional (as it was in this case), or spiritual. The pain of loss can be as devastating as the pain that is associated with physical injury. Dreams such as this one can help heal wounds that might otherwise cripple the dreamer on an emotional or spiritual level.

Dream 39:
Psalm 91

Dreamer: A mother in Georgia

Source: God

Color: Muted (as reported by dreamer); most likely normal colors

Dream Category: Intercessory dream

Dream: In my dream, I heard a voice speak to me and say, "Satan is trying to destroy your children. Pray Psalm 91 over your children."

Dreamer's Understanding/Interpretation: I knew I needed to pray Psalm 91 over my children's lives.

Author's Spirit-Led Interpretation: This is a direction from the Lord to intercede for your children and pray the promises of Psalm 91 over their lives.

Impact/Outcome: My two children had both been having close calls with death for several weeks. These experiences were ongoing and seemed to have been coming one right after another. After I had the dream and I began praying Psalm 91 over the lives of my children, the close calls ceased. I have continued to pray Psalm 91 over my children's lives, though they are now adults.

Primary Metaphor(s):

Voice—voice of the Lord

Lesson: This dream is straightforward and needs little interpretation. It is a directive from the Lord to a mother to intercede for the lives of her children. Remember that while dreams are metaphorical and often contain symbols that need interpretation, the Lord can also speak very directly in what we would call a dream. In a dream/vision such as this, the voice that is heard is more similar to a prophetic declaration than what we would normally associate with a dream. In these cases, the weight that such a prophetic word carries is often more significant than it would have carried if it was coming from and filtered through a fellow believer. This is true because the word is received as coming directly from the Lord to the recipient.

Dream 40:
A Dream Come True

 (Use the QR code to hear the dreamer give more details about the dream and its significance. If you do not have access to a QR code reader, the Web site associated with this dream is listed in the INDEX.)

Dreamer: A woman in Hawaii, but she was in California at the time of the dream

Source: God

Color: Color

Dream Category: Direction dream

Dream: In my dream, I was on a beach that had a beautiful span of short grass with palm trees on the edge of the lava-rock shelf overlooking the ocean with a small stretch of sand. It was so real. A few months later, in September of 1992, I had the same dream again.

Dreamer's Understanding/Interpretation: I felt as if the dream had to do with a place we were supposed to live.

Author's Spirit-Led Interpretation: The Lord is calling you to a place of peace from which your ministry will have a significant impact. It is possible that this is a physical, geographical location.

Impact/Outcome: A few weeks after I had the dream for the second time, a friend called my husband and asked whether he was working, and my husband informed him that he was not at that time. The friend proceeded to tell my husband about how Hurricane Iniki (which struck on September 11, 1992) had devastated the island of Kauai and how experienced roofers were needed on the island to reconstruct the roofs of the houses and buildings. We flew to Kauai on October 4, 1992, and lived in Kapaa (on the east side of the island) for nine months. We then moved to Omao, on the south side of the island. As we were driving to the beach, about ten minutes from where we lived, we passed a restaurant, and I saw the scene from my dream. I shouted for my husband to stop the car. God had confirmed that this was the place that He wanted us to be.

Primary Metaphor(s):

Ocean—large impact, masses of people

Grass and palm trees—a place of peace

Lesson: As has been mentioned, dreams often have multiple interpretations. It is unlikely that even an individual experienced in biblical dream interpretation would interpret this dream as a instruction to move to Hawaii (unless they had heard a clear word from the Holy Spirit). However, that does not mean this is not a direction dream. The dream indicates that the place from which the couple would minister would be a place of peace and that they would have an impact on many people. On another level, however, the dream gives a geographic assignment. Even if the direction to move was not clear at the time of the dream (although in this case, the dreamer felt that in her spirit), it does later serve as a confirmation that they were in the correct physical location. At the time of this book's publication, this couple remains on the island of Kauai, ministering to the people there.

Dream 41:
A Single Season Could Take Nine Years

Dreamer: A woman in Singapore

Source: The enemy/God

Color: Black-and-white/color

Dream Category: Dark/Deliverance dream

Dream: When I was fourteen years old, I dozed off while studying and instantly felt as if my soul had separated from my body. I was sinking deep down into a dark abyss that felt devoid of anything and everything. It was an absolute nothingness. There was nothing I could do. Then I heard a crackling voice call out my full name and say, "I am going to make you fall. Don't think you can do anything great for the Almighty. I will make sure you fall and never stand again!" When I woke up, it felt like I had been in the dream for nine years.

At the age of nineteen, I had a dream that seemed connected to me. I was outside a club, in the line to enter. I was almost at the entrance when someone tapped on my shoulder and said, "I have something important to tell you." After a moment of hesitation, I followed her and the setting changed. I was suddenly in a regular apartment in Singapore, and the person pulled out a list that described things that were going to happen. I only remember that the last item on the list was "darkness." I looked to the right, and I saw a zombie kneeling on the floor. It was dormant. I prayed and attempted to get it to leave, but it wouldn't budge. At that point, a leader appeared, and as he arrived, I saw waves of similar but smaller zombies coming toward us. The three of us started praying and commanding them to go.

Dreamer's Understanding/Interpretation: I felt after the first dream that I was about to go through a difficult season that would last nine years. In the second dream, I felt that I was waiting to step into my calling, but that I was waiting in the wrong place. I felt that the Lord would lead me to the right place for a breakthrough.

Author's Spirit-Led Interpretation: The enemy is intent on destroying the call of God on both you and your life, but the Lord is going to remove you from the place where the world is enticing you and take you to a place where you can be free from the enemy's oppression and live out your spiritual destiny. The season of transition in your life may take some time to come to pass.

Impact/Outcome: I reached the lowest point in my life at the age of twenty-one. I fell into deep depression. About that same time, I realized that the two dreams were connected, and that since the first one had occurred at the age of fourteen, my breakthrough should come by the age of twenty-three. I felt that I needed to take some time off work to sort out my life. I ended up feeling called to leave Singapore, and I applied for a passport, which was issued on my twenty-third birthday—nine years after the first dream. I am now living in Hong Kong, working in a ministry and teaching English to children. The understanding of the dream that came at age twenty-one pulled me out of the darkness and propelled me into God's purpose for my life.

Primary Metaphor(s):

Zombies—demonic attackers

Person with list—an angel

Leader—God

Lesson: The first of these dreams is a dark dream sent by the enemy to destroy the life of the dreamer and leave her with a sense of hopelessness. The second provides the hope to overcome the darkness thrust upon the dreamer after the first dream. Notice the time that it took for this dream to have a significant impact upon the dreamer. At the time of the dreams, little to no understanding came. It was not until years later (seven years from the first dream, and two years from the second) that the understanding of the dream clicked and made its impact. Some dreams can take even more time to come to pass or to impact the dreamer's life (for example, the dreams that Joseph had in Genesis 37). Without understanding, a dream can either impact the dreamer in a negative way or cause him or her to remain unsettled, creating a deep desire to search out the true interpretation.

Although this dream took some time to come to fruition, having had it and coming to an understanding of it were vital for the dreamer to overcome the dark place in her life. Notice that the dreamer indicated that she had been at the lowest point of her life at the age of twenty-one, but that it was also at that time when she realized the full connection between the dreams and she found hope that in just a short period of time, things would change. This is a beautiful illustration of the principle previously mentioned, that what the enemy intends for evil, God will turn and use for good (see Genesis 50:20).

Dream Stories by Michael B. French

Dream 42:
The Truth About My Father and My Grief

 *(Use the QR code to hear the dreamer give more details about the dream and its significance. If you do not have access to a QR code reader, the Web site associated with this dream is listed in the INDEX.)*

Dreamer: A woman in Florida

Source: God

Color: Full colors

Dream Category: Healing dream

Dream: My mother and I are standing by an airplane waiting for passengers to disembark. We know that my father is on the plane and that he is finally coming home. I ask my mother whether I should call him Dad or Daddy, and she says that he would be glad either way. Suddenly we see him behind a stream of people. He is small and looks fragile. He has broken ribs and is bruised on his upper body. He is injured, so I can't hug him very hard. In the next scene, I'm on the lawn behind my Swedish grandparents' home. I see a large military helicopter. My dad, some other person I don't know, and I are all walking around. When I ask Dad why he didn't come home, he says he flew more missions so that he could get a domestic assignment and then come home to me. I start to cry and tell him that I had needed him and he wasn't there. I'm not sure whether he hugged me. In the next scene, my grandmother, my cousin (who is like a sister to me), and I are in one of the guest rooms. I'm sitting on the bed crying, and they are trying to comfort me. They both know that my dad has returned. I tell them that I've dreamt of this day my entire life. Suddenly I don't feel well, and I go to the bathroom, where I start to pull something out of my mouth. I keep pulling, and out comes something very long, all the way up from my stomach. Finally, it is all out, and I take it over to my cousin, who explains that it is fat. It crumbles and melts as it comes out, and I feel embarrassed and return to the bathroom to wash it away.

Dreamer's Understanding/Interpretation: God used this dream to tell me that my father didn't fly extra missions to get medals, but to come home to me sooner.

Author's Spirit-Led Interpretation: This dream is to let you know that your father loves you, even though there has been hurt and pain that has made it difficult to understand his love. God is removing the grief that was intended to destroy you, and He is beginning a cleansing work that will set you free.

Impact/Outcome: My father was killed in Vietnam in 1967, when I was a small child. In the dream, I was in the same room where my mother stayed and grieved when she learned that my father had been killed. After this dream, I no longer held my mother's offense/grudge against my father. She had grown angry at his career choice, and she resented the posthumous medals he had received. I knew from that point on that he had loved me. Only my mother received support in her grief when he died, not my brother or me. The dream also validated the fact that I had lost someone important to me and that it was okay for me to mourn my loss.

Primary Metaphor(s):

Broken ribs—pain

Bathroom—a place to get cleaned up, deliverance

Fat—unhealthy emotions that have built up over time

Lesson: When interpreting a dream such as this, it is important to remember that unless the Lord gives you specific understanding, it may be difficult to know whether the dream is about the dreamer's natural father or their heavenly Father. By using language in the interpretation that allows the dreamer to make this application herself, it prevents an assumption from impacting the significance of what the Holy Spirit is saying.

Elements in dreams tend to take their meaning from their actual function or usage. In this case, one of the keys to understanding the emotional pain that is at the heart of the dream is the fact that it is the dreamer's father's ribs that are broken and bruised. Ribs are designed to protect the heart (they are often synonymous with emotions), and the capacity for them to do so in this case has been compromised. This is also a good indication that the dream may be about the dreamer's natural father and not her heavenly Father.

Dream Stories by Michael B. French

Dream 43: Don

Dreamer: A female missionary in Honduras

Source: God

Color: Full colors

Dream Category: Warning dream

Dream: This dream took place in the inner yard at our farm in Honduras. My husband and I were standing outside, and he was doing pool maintenance. Suddenly, out of nowhere, there was a little Honduran girl who was maybe three or four years old. She went up to my husband, and I heard him say, "*No, papi,*" and then she walked away. I saw sadness on her face, and I wondered why my husband hadn't helped her, but I thought he must have had a good reason. Then there was another child, and again he said no. More people and animals began to show up all over our yard, and all of them wanted either money or food. I knew that we were not supposed to give it to them. I even saw a little child coming up out of the ground like an elderly turtle, and I immediately threw some liquid from a pan at him to get him to go away. Next, I saw a line of dogs along the wall of our property, and the gate was open. I looked at the wall and said to myself, *So, that's why we have a wall.* I woke up.

Dreamer's Understanding/Interpretation: This dream was partially literal about whom we let into the inner sanctuary of our home, as opposed to the outer fields. Also, God was warning me that I needed to set boundaries and not take on more than what He had given me to do. We were also to take care of our own spiritual life as a priority.

Author's Spirit-Led Interpretation: You have open doors in your ministry that have allowed people to try to take advantage of your compassion and drain you. It is important to maintain your own spiritual relationship with the Lord and guard yourself against the ways in which the enemy may try to take advantage of you in the work that you do. God has set a hedge of protection in place around you, but you must keep the doors closed that would allow the enemy access.

Impact/Outcome: I immediately started to pay more attention to my personal secret place with God, but I came to realize that the dream also had practical application. We literally have a farm in Honduras where we grow fruits and vegetables to feed the hungry. We began to see more and more people coming to our farm, both for help and for recreation. The dream helped me to recognize the need for boundaries and to become more comfortable with those we had to set in order to keep ourselves safe and sane.

Primary Metaphor(s):

Inner yard—secret place

Pool maintenance—maintaining spiritual things

"*No, papi*"—appropriate boundaries

Open gate—an open door through which the enemy can enter

Lesson: This dream is a great illustration of how layers of meaning can exist in a single dream. Here, the dream is initially understood, and rightly so, as a warning that the dreamer needs to pay attention to her quiet time or her secret place with the Lord. Bodies of water, whether natural or manmade (such as swimming pools), are often representative of a place where a person can get into the things of the Spirit. Water is frequently associated both with the Word of God and with the Holy Spirit, and a swimming pool, such as the one in this dream, is a place for a person to dive in to the water (either the Word or the Spirit, both of which represent the things of God). Here, maintenance is being done on the pool, thus indicating that there is work that needs to be done to keep the place where the dreamer gets into the Word/Spirit functional.

As time passes, the second layer of understanding concerning this dream becomes more recognizable. Not only does the dreamer need to guard her heart to maintain a closeness of relationship to the Lord, but there are practical things that need to be guarded, as well. In a mission environment, where great needs exist and individuals are attempting to meet them, it is easy to become overwhelmed. The warning that people would try to take advantage of the compassion of the dreamer does not necessarily indicate a danger of physical harm, but the presence of both the fence and the guard dogs lined up on it does indicate the need for protection on a natural level. The elderly turtle coming out of the ground indicates that the issue has been around for a long season, but that now is the time to deal with it. Nothing in the dream indicates that the dreamer should stop the work that she is doing, but it does indicate that there are good reasons to limit access to the dreamer's private life and personal space.

Dream 44:
God Dream as a Child

Dreamer: A four-year-old girl in Ohio

Source: God

Color: Colors

Dream Category: Calling dream

Dream: I was lying in bed next to the window, and my spirit left my body and went through the window and up to the top of the house. I was dressed in a white gown, like an angel flying around the middle of the top of the house. It was dark outside, and as I looked around I saw trees, hillsides, and houses close by and in the distance. I knew that if I flew away from the house, I would get lost. I flew around the house a few times and then back through the window and into my body.

Dreamer's Understanding/Interpretation: I did not understand the dream at the time, but I never forgot it. As I matured, I came to believe that the Lord was going to use me to be a watchman over my family.

Author's Spirit-Led Interpretation: This interpretation is presented for the benefit of the adult recalling the dream from her childhood. The Lord has had His hand upon you since you were a child. There has been a prophetic gift in operation in your life since you were little, though there have been times when it was confusing and you knew you could not show it to the world. Rather, you believed that you had to keep it close (you used it first in relation to your family and those near you) and learn to walk in it.

Impact/Outcome: After I grew up and began to understand the dream, I knew it was a huge responsibility, and it caused me to pray and intercede more and ask the Lord for more clarity in knowing His voice and guidance.

Primary Metaphor(s):

Flying—moving higher into spiritual things, often a symbol of a prophetic gifting

Child's house—one's own family or life

Lesson: This lesson should be prefaced with a reminder that many people have dreams as children, the memory of which lingers vividly into their adult lives. While the dream may not be understood by the child, God knows the right time for an interpretation to have the most impact. His patience in waiting for us to hear His voice is evidenced by such dreams.

The greatest lesson that can be learned from this dream is never to take for granted the dreams of a small child. God is not a respecter of persons when it comes to age. He will speak to a four-year-old, a forty-year-old, or a ninety-four-year-old. We must learn not to destroy the gifts of God in our children. It can be so easy for a parent to assume that an experience such as this is the product of an overactive imagination or that the "monster under the bed" is nothing more than a fearful desire for Mom and Dad to let them sleep in their parents' room. While that may at times be the case, it is also possible that it is a spiritual experience or that the "monster" is a demonic assault that needs to be overcome. Jeremiah was called before he was formed in his mother's womb, and John the Baptist leapt in utero when he spiritually discerned the presence of the Messiah in the belly of another. Instead of assuming that it is merely the product of a child's imagination, it is time that we begin to expect spiritual experiences and encourage our children to grow up expecting them, as well.

It should be noted here that this dream involves an experience that can be challenging for some Christians to understand, let alone accept. The reference to the phrase "my spirit left my body" needs some explanation. There are many experiences that have a biblical basis but that have been counterfeited and corrupted by the enemy. For example, Paul seems to reference this type of experience when he declares, "I know a man in Christ who fourteen years ago was caught up to the third heaven. Whether it was in the body or out of the body I do not know—God knows" (2 Corinthians 12:2, NIV). In addition, John seems to reference such experiences in the book of Revelation. However, due to New Age practices such as astral projection, the Church has steered clear of such experiences. The safest approach for a Christian is never to seek out such experiences, yet to recognize that when they are initiated by God, there is no biblical evidence to suggest that they are inappropriate.

Dream 45:
Saying Good-Bye

Dreamer: A woman in Alabama

Source: The enemy/God

Color: Black and white/colors

Dream Category: Dark/Healing dream

Dream: My dream was devoid of color. In it, my mother, who had died after a brief bout with cancer, came to me, and we were walking down a dirt road. I told her how much I loved her and thanked her for everything she had ever done for me and for loving me. As we continued to walk down the road, she said to me, "You know I will be leaving you again. I love you, too." Then she turned to me, and her eyes became the most brilliant color of gold that I had ever seen. She smiled and walked on down the dirt road until she faded away into the air. I will never forget the color of her eyes as she said good-bye. When I awoke from the dream, I felt tremendous peace.

Dreamer's Understanding/Interpretation: I had been begging the Lord to send my mother back to me so that I could tell her all the unspoken things I hadn't told her before she died. I felt this dream was sent to give me a chance to say good-bye to my mother.

Author's Spirit-Led Interpretation: This is a dream from the enemy that was sent to draw you into a place of dependence upon experiential comfort; however, because of the purity and innocence of your petitions, the Lord intervened and gave you the peace for which you were searching.

Impact/Outcome: I had entered into a place of deep depression over the loss of my mother. It was out of this depression that I was begging the Lord to send her back to for me to see her one more time again. During the dream, I felt such love for my mother, and when I woke up I felt peace knowing that I'd had the chance to say good-bye.

Primary Metaphor(s):

Mother—literal in this case

Conversation—giving voice to unspoken things

Gold—refining, purification, holiness

Eyes—revelation, ability to see in the Spirit

Lesson: The black-and-white context of this dream points to the fact that it was initially from the enemy. Note that this dream was the result of a soul crying out of a place of deep depression, and it does not represent the typical way that the Lord would relate to such a state of mind, also indicating that the dream was not from Him. Because the repeated requests to see her deceased mother again came out of innocence, this was not the same as necromancy (a knowing and intentional seeking out of the dead, usually for information).

While the enemy sent this dream to snare the dreamer in a trap that would have perpetuated the depression when her mother had to leave her again, the Lord intervened and inserted His message into the dream (at this point, the dream became a dream from God). When the color appeared in the dream—the beautiful golden eyes—the metaphor used was the message from God that brings peace. Gold is something that gains value from being refined and purified, just as God did with this dream. The eyes speak to the ability to see, particularly to see in the Spirit. God purified the dream and released peace for the dreamer to see her release as coming from the Spirit of God and not from her petition for her mother to appear to her. In this way, the departure of the dreamer's mother in the dream did not lead her to return to a place of depression at the conclusion of a temporary experience. Instead, the dream led to lasting release, because the Spirit of the Lord intervened and ministered peace to the dreamer.

This dream falls into the same category as the dream entitled "God Dream as a Child," which involves an encounter that should not be pursued (encountering the dreamer's mother after begging for this to occur), but it is not beyond the realm of biblically acceptable phenomena if it is initiated by God. To fully address this particular issue is, however, beyond the scope of this book.

Dream 46: Neglected/Forgotten Pet

Dreamer: A woman in Scotland

Source: God

Color: Full colors

Dream Category: Calling dream

Dream: In the dream, I am in my house and I suddenly remember that I have a young pet (it is either a puppy or a kitten), but that I forgot I had it, and now I wonder whether it is still alive. I had forgotten to take care of it (giving it food, water, and care). I begin to feel terrible about this, that I had neglected something so precious. I then begin to search the house for my young pet, as well as try to find some food and water to give it. I hope and pray it is not too late and that I will find my pet still alive.

Dreamer's Understanding/Interpretation: I did not understand the dream, but I had it repeatedly for almost a year. It reached a point that when I would fall asleep and the dream started, I would actually think in the dream, *Oh no, here is that dream AGAIN!*

Author's Spirit-Led Interpretation: God has given you a gift, but you have neglected to use it and take care of it, and now it is almost ready to fade away.

Impact/Outcome: This dream was a wake-up call for me to repent and begin to function in what God was calling me to do. For some time, God had been speaking to me that He had given me a teaching gift. Because I was intimidated, I did nothing about it. After the dream was interpreted for me, I asked God to confirm whether the dream was about that particular gift, and within an hour I received three invitations to speak and teach at various places. Since then, I have continued to accept invitations to teach and I have actually begun to teach on biblical dream interpretation with Streams Ministries International.

Primary Metaphor(s):

Pet—something precious, a gift

Neglect—literal, the gift has not been cared for or used

Search—encouragement to seek out and care for the gift

Lesson: While the gifts and callings of God are irrevocable (see Romans 11:29), this does not mean that those who receive them should ignore them. This dream is a beautiful example of how God loves us enough to remind us of our calling and purpose in order that we might not squander what we have been given. He uses imagery here, such as the puppy/kitten, that evokes emotions and causes the dreamer to understand the pain brought about by neglecting a living thing that is so precious. The imagery is beautiful, because our gifts are also living, powerful, and precious.

The repetitive nature of this dream indicates the emphasis that God is placing on saving the gift that has been given to the dreamer. The nature of the dream creates a spiritual irritation, much like the sound of fingernails being scraped across a chalkboard. This serves to unsettle the dreamer each time the dream is repeated, not in a harmful fashion, but rather to drive the dreamer to come to an understanding of the dream and to recognize what she has been neglecting. In this way, the irritation also becomes a metaphor, and like an itch that needs to be scratched, this dream cries out for a response.

Dream Stories by Michael B. French

Dream 47:
A New Name

Dreamer: A woman in Hong Kong

Source: God

Color: Full colors

Dream Category: Self-condition dream

Dream: I am in a building with windows from floor to ceiling. It seems to be an airport, and it is a sunny day. In the dream, I am wearing a one-piece, long white dress, and I am walking toward a crowd at the waiting area in front of the departure gate. A group of people is coming from an airplane at one of the gates, and I see a foreigner among them who catches my attention. I know I need to follow him, even though I have never met him before. I don't ask myself why; I just follow. We make eye contact, and he twitches his head and raises his eyebrows, signaling for me to follow. He walks very fast and has a briefcase with him. He has a birthmark on his left temple and is similar in height and body size to Michael J. Fox, the former television actor.

The man leads me into an open café or sitting area on the same level of the building. The café's table is situated between two, tall, C-shaped mud-brown sofas. The foreigner and I sit on one side, and there is another person on the opposite side. The other man is wearing a black suit and he greets the foreigner with respect, but I cannot see his face. The foreigner opens a file from his briefcase, and when I see it, I think to myself, *Oh no!* There are four small, green, government-style envelopes that each have a blue handwritten signature on them. I do not know what is inside the envelopes, but I am certain that it is not good at all (perhaps it relates to forbidden contracts, my debts, or other illegal/troubling things). I am very afraid when I see the files and I begin to worry about my entire life, both my past mistakes and the things I might do wrong in the future. I feel that the two are going to judge me, and if they do I would die.

I try to sneak behind the foreigner's back and hide. When I do, he stops me, and I hear him speak in my mind, *Kayla . . .* , but I don't know what else he says because I am thinking about the fact that my name is not Kayla. I feel as if he is trying to tell me to be still. The voice is very intense, and so I obey. I can hear a little of the conversation between the two men, and I remember the foreigner saying something like, "I know she signed an agreement with you, but . . ." Then the sound seems to be muted. I realize that whoever has arranged this meeting must love me so much that they have arranged to pay off everything and help me out of the unjust deals I had made. I feel like Cinderella and wonder how someone can love me that much.

Dreamer's Understanding/Interpretation: God paid all my debts and has cleared all the bad things from my past.

Author's Spirit-Led Interpretation: God has chosen you. He has given you a new name and a new identity, which separates you from the mistakes of your past. He has and He will continue to protect you from the plans of the enemy. This is a time and a place in your life for new vision to come forth and launch you into your destiny.

Impact/Outcome: This dream caused such intense emotion and the strong feeling of being loved. It felt like a fairy tale. After a decade, a dream teacher helped me to understand the name I had been called in the dream and its meaning. I was deeply moved by receiving a new name and I felt that things were changing in my life at a quantum level. I have actually changed my name and begun to use the name Kayla as a part of my real name.

Primary Metaphor(s):

Kayla—this name means "pure"

New name—new identity

Files—record of the past, one's history

Foreigner (Michael J. Fox)—Jesus; the name "Michael" means "Who is like God?" with the middle initial of *J* for *Jesus*

Lesson: The core of this dream was clear to the dreamer. Her life had been changed, and she was set free from her past, but a single element remained unclear: In situations such as this, the Lord sometimes conceals or veils a portion of the dream until the right timing for it to be revealed. Here, it is the new name. It was ten years after she had the dream before her new name was fully understood and embraced. This, too, is a metaphor. Receiving Jesus may cancel our past debts, but we must then learn to walk in and fully embrace the new identity we have been given.

When our history is used by the enemy in an effort to destroy us, God has many ways in which He encourages us to overcome. One such way is illustrated by this dream, as it clarifies for the dreamer that her condition was no longer based upon what the enemy accused her of, but upon how God saw her. Self-condition dreams can point out issues in a dreamer's life that need to be corrected, but they can also identify areas in which the dreamers need to see themselves as God does.

Dream 48: Minefield

(Use the QR code to hear the dreamer give more details about the dream and its significance. If you do not have access to a QR code reader, the Web site associated with this dream is listed in the INDEX.)

Dreamer: A soldier on the battlefield during the Korean War, as recounted by his son

Source: God

Color: Colors

Dream Category: Prophetic dream

Dream: In my dream, I was on the battlefield in the exact area where my unit had been positioned at the time of the dream. I was walking across an open area and I saw that there were land mines everywhere. As I walked around, I saw exactly where each land mine had been positioned.

Dreamer's Understanding/Interpretation: I felt that the dream was showing me where the land mines were located on the battlefield.

Author's Spirit-Led Interpretation: There are a number of hidden dangers in your path, but God is providing a way of escape. Because this dream took place on the battlefield in the midst of a war, it is also prophetic and may reveal where the actual land mines are on the battlefield.

Impact/Outcome: Sometime between 1950 and 1952, my father was serving in the United States military. This was during the Korean War. His unit was ordered to cross an area that had previously been controlled by the enemy and was known to be heavily land mined. Significant casualties were expected. The night before they were to cross the area, my father had this dream. The next morning, he approached his commanding officer about the dream, and the commander decided it was worth taking seriously. He sent my father with the Explosive Ordinance Disposal specialists, and together they were able to locate and disarm the very same mines my father had seen in the dream. The entire unit crossed the area safely without a single casualty. Many lives were saved, potentially including my father's. I think about the fact that I might never have been born, had the Lord not given my father this dream.

Primary Metaphor(s):

Land mines—hidden dangers

Lesson: This is one of those dreams that could have easily been brushed off as being caused by the existing circumstances or brought out from fear of the assignment that had been given to this soldier and his unit. Instead, the dreamer took the dream seriously and acted on it as if it was a revelation from God. Because dreams can have multiple layers of meaning, the spiritual interpretation that there are hidden dangers may also be directly applicable to the dreamer's life, but to have ignored the prophetic warning that the dream provided would have been devastating. It is important to learn that we must never be satisfied with a surface or a soulish understanding of a dream. This dream is yet another reminder that we cannot become dependent upon a dictionary-style interpretation of symbols to provide the full meaning of a Spirit-inspired dream.

Additionally, this dream provides a wonderful illustration of the difference between interpretation and application. The interpretation of a dream involves understanding what the dream means. Here, the interpretation brings understanding that there is something hidden, but God will reveal it and provide protection. Application involves understanding how the interpretation can be used to make a difference in the dreamer's life. In this situation, the dreamer identified the literal application of the dream from the context of its relationship to his present situation. While the application was very easy to identify in this particular dream, this aspect of biblical dream interpretation can often be one of the most challenging.

Dream Stories by Michael B. French

Dream 49:
An Office at Jacksonville

Dreamer: The author of this book (Michael B. French)

Source: God

Color: Vivid colors

Dream Category: Direction/Prophetic/Courage dream

Dream: In my dream, I left the church and went to a meeting at Jacksonville State University (where I literally had attended college and had served as the student government president) to observe a presidential search committee that was seeking someone to fill the vacancy of university president. The committee chairman suddenly began to interview me for the job, and then he started handing me gifts that I would need for my new office. A woman at the other end of the table objected and said that those gifts were for the new president, to which the chairman replied, "Yes, but you should already know that Michael is the new president." I woke up. When I went back to sleep, the dream picked up in my new office as president of the university. I was welcoming people from the church and other ministries into my new office and surprising them by telling them it was mine and that I had left my previous job and was now serving as the president of the university. I woke up. When I went back to sleep, the dream picked up again with me admiring the large, beautiful bathroom that my new office contained and feeling very excited about being able to use it.

Dreamer's Understanding/Interpretation: It was my sense that the interpretation to my dream was that God was moving me into a new position suddenly and that He was giving me the gifts needed to do it.

Author's Spirit-Led Interpretation: God is moving you into a new position and providing what is needed to fill it. While there may be those who don't understand what is happening, God will reassure them. The suddenness of the move will be surprising and unexpected, but there will be joy in releasing those things that have weighed you down.

Impact/Outcome: I pastored the Bridge Birmingham for seventeen years. Within three weeks of having this dream, I gave up my pastoral role and our church merged with another body of believers, so that I could take on the full-time position of leading Patria Ministries (a family of churches, ministries, and Kingdom-minded businesses; see www.patriamin.com). I was able to turn over some of the most challenging tasks I had been carrying and focus instead on what God had given me to do.

Two years prior to this dream, one of my spiritual fathers and mentor, John Paul Jackson, had blessed me and commissioned me to begin Patria Ministries, but I had still been working at it in a part-time fashion. When I moved into a full-time role, the growth of that ministry became exponential.

Primary Metaphor(s):

Jacksonville State University—a place of training (in this case, received from John Paul Jackson)

President—position of authority

New office—new position

Bathroom—a place to release toxins and get cleaned up

Lesson: Dreams often fit into more than one category, something that is very true in this case. This dream clearly gave directions for where I was to go and the timing in which it was supposed to occur. However, the dream also provided me with the courage to take those steps in the time frame the dream indicated. Finally, there were elements of the dream that were very directly prophetic, such as the fact that it indicated that when I stepped into the proper place as president of the ministry, I would be able to welcome many to join, an element fulfilled by the increased growth of the ministry when I moved into leading it on a full-time basis. Though the dreams that follow have been placed into various categories to help bring understanding to them, never attempt to limit how God uses a dream or what He might be saying through it.

Recognize that many things can indicate the significance of a dream. Be sure to pay attention when a dream feels significant. It may be that you don't normally remember your dreams, but you can't forget the one you had last night, or perhaps you have the dream repeatedly. Sometimes the indicator is the emotional weight you feel in the dream or after you wake up, and other times, it may be how real the dream seemed as you were in it. When a dream seems significant, it probably is—so don't ignore it; seek the Lord for wisdom on what He is saying through it.

Dream Stories by Michael B. French

Dream 50:
1987 Market Crash

 *(Use the QR code to hear the dreamer give more details about the dream and its significance. If you do not have access to a QR code reader, the Web site associated with this dream is listed in the INDEX.)*

Dreamer: A man in Northern Ireland

Source: God

Color: Full colors

Dream Category: Prophetic/Warning dream

Dream: I had this dream in May 1987. There are three scenes in this dream:

In each scene, I'm standing in the same place and the setting is the same. I'm standing on a mountain watching these events unfold before me and below me. There is a river running from north to south. I just know this. The river is depicted as flowing from right to left. (All the action occurs from right to left) Three-quarters of the way along the riverbank to my left is a large castle. This castle obscures my vision of the part of the river behind it.

In the first scene, Canadian geese fly along the river from right to left. They then disappear, exiting stage left.

In the second scene, a flock of flamingos suddenly lift off from the river, again flying from right to left. One of them has a large bag of money tied to its left leg (the sort of thing you'd see in a children's cartoon). On the bag is a £ or $ symbol. These birds all fly into the castle and disappear.

In the third scene, a ferocious black bear suddenly appears, thrashing its way along the river at enormous speed. This bear brings a great sense of danger, fear, and panic. Again, the action takes place from right to left. When the bear arrives, I immediately feel I need to get my family to a place of safety. At one point, the bear disappears behind the castle. I don't know whether the bear is confined to the river or if it has emerged from the river and is now attacking the castle.

At this point, I am shown two Christians I know who were also financial consultants. They have more money than me, around forty million pounds, in their portfolios. When they appear, the scene becomes darker. A voice tells me not to get involved with these men.

Dreamer's Understanding/Interpretation: I eventually figured out scenes two and three of the dream, which told me to be nervous and to quickly respond like the flamingos did. I was to take my clients' money out of the financial markets, because a dangerous bear market was suddenly coming. I didn't understand scene one until a month or so after the 1987 market crash on October 19th. Scene one gave me the timing (October, which is the time when Canadian geese fly south). I understood the full interpretation to be: In October, I was to remove my money from the markets and put it into the safety of the Building Society, because a sudden bear market that would cause fear and panic was coming.

Sadly, I didn't press in to understand scene one in time.

Author's Spirit-Led Interpretation: There is a season coming in which you need to move quickly and exercise caution with regard to your finances, because a sudden and ferocious bear market is coming. Do not get involved with the two people you saw at the end of your dream.

Impact/Outcome: I learned that I should have pressed in to understand the full dream, as I missed its timing. When I shared my concerns with others, few listened, because I could not be specific with regard to the timing of my warning. I ended up leaving the firm I was with, and a friend and I opened our own privately managed fund. My partner and I had convinced our own clients to come out of the market, and we had their money safely in a bank account awaiting a strategy when the October 1987 stock market crash happened. As a financial consultant, perhaps I could have helped still others to move their investments out of the stock market and into the Building Society managed funds before the market crashed. This could have been done without requiring much faith/risk on the part of both consultants or their clients and at no cost to either. But I disregarded God's warning about the two financial consultants and I joined forces with them after the crash. I ended up wasting a lot of time and money. I have been convicted in paying deeper attention to my current dreams. I also know that although I thought God was going to show me how to get into and out of the financial markets, He was actually calling me to leave the investment world altogether, because He had different plans for my life.

Primary Metaphor(s):

Canadian geese migration—timing, when the geese fly south

Castle—symbol of the Building Society in the United Kingdom (which was safer and stronger than banks at the time of the dream)

Flamingos—being easily startled and having a quick reaction time

Bear—a financial market when share prices fall

Lesson: There several lessons that can learned from this dream:

This dream represents a significant need for dreamers to take their dreams seriously and seek full understanding of their meaning from the Lord. By valuing both the dream and the interpretation, the fullness of what God is saying through them can be brought to a place of application to our lives and not be left hanging with an incomplete or partial understanding.

This dream is a wonderful illustration of how the meaning of dream symbols can change from dream to dream and from culture to culture. A castle might frequently be seen as a stronghold, or even a place of authority, but at this time and in this culture, it was widely known to represent a specific thing—the Building Society. To simply apply an acceptable and common meaning to this particular symbol would have hindered a complete understanding of the dream. However, the understanding might not have been completely lost, because the Building Society was also a safe stronghold for finances at that time.

We can also learn that there is a time and a place to share what we have heard from God and a time and a place to simply pray. The dreamer did not have the favor with others that would allow him to be heard, and because he lacked a complete understanding of the timing, it was even more difficult for that favor to be established. In this case, the dreamer and those who trusted him could respond, but the only impact that he could have on others was to pray.

Finally, there is a great lesson here concerning how God can speak in many different ways to provide the meaning of a dream symbol. As the dreamer recounted this dream and how he came to an understanding of it, three very distinct methods of interpreting the individual metaphors emerged. The July 1987 issue of *Prophecy Today* ran an article on greed and a possible downturn in the stock market that caught the dreamer's attention about the same time as he heard a prophetic word on the same subject. These things confirmed that the "bear" in his dream symbolized a bear market. The dreamer was later watching a nature television show and he saw a group of thousands of flamingos take flight at a sudden disturbance, providing understanding of this symbol in his dream. Although it did not come until after the market crash, an understanding of the Canadian geese came from a conversation with an American from New Hampshire with whom he shared the dream and learned that geese fill the sky each year in October as they begin their migration south for the winter.

Dream 51:
Surveying the Land with Jesus

Dreamer: A woman in Ohio

Source: God

Color: Full colors

Dream Category: Flushing dream

Dream: I dreamed that I walked with a man and went to the top of a hill on my family's land where I grew up. In the wooded area at the top of the hill, there was a strip that had been cleared of the old trees, and some new trees had been planted and were growing. The new trees were a beautiful pink and a pale green, and yet the colors were so vibrant and beautiful that I was in awe. I wondered about them, as I had never seen these colors before, let alone on trees. The man walking with me seemed to show me this scene, then he gave me a hug that flooded me with overwhelming love. I said that I had to get back to my husband, and then I woke up.

Dreamer's Understanding/Interpretation: I sensed that the new trees were good things that had been planted in my family. The old trees were removed (like removing curses), and the new ones were passing down blessings. The man walking with me and hugging me represented Jesus and the fact that He was with me throughout my journey.

Author's Spirit-Led Interpretation: There are some issues in your family line that you may not be aware of that have resulted in a generational curse. The Lord is removing the curse and replacing it with fresh, new things that will bring forth a blessing.

Impact/Outcome: I felt cleansing during the dream and a flood of love. It was overwhelming! I felt that family curses were cut off and blessings were brought down as the love of Jesus flooded through me.

Primary Metaphor(s):

Family land—family line, inheritance

Trees—leaders, in this case family leaders

Pink and pale green—pastel colors that represent love and growth that has not yet reached full maturity

Lesson: While this dream could be classified as a deliverance dream, because generational curses were broken off as a result of it, it is much more akin to a flushing dream. Flushing dreams are God's way of cleansing the dreamer from any things the enemy has used to affect his or her life. In many cases, the dream would arise from issues that have arisen in the life of the dreamer, oftentimes involving things without the dreamer having full awareness of or even a responsibility for on a personal level (that is, they did nothing that caused such things to touch their lives).

Trees often represent leaders. The basis for this understanding of the metaphor is taken from the Scriptures, specifically Daniel 4, in which Nebuchadnezzar is depicted as a great tree in the dream. Dreams that return us to a childhood or family home are frequently related to family issues, and in this dream, the fact that the old trees have been removed shows that there is evidence that something related to those family leaders needs to be removed from the dreamer's life.

While colors have great meaning in dreams, the nature of the colors is also important. As has previously been discussed, muted colors are often representative of a dream that the enemy has planted; however, it is important to distinguish between *muted* colors and *pastel* colors. Pastels are full and complete colors, even though they are a lighter shade of the primary color to which they relate. In this case, pale green is obvious, and pink is a pastel/lighter shade of red. Because red can represent love and green can represent growth, the lighter shades depicted in this full-color dream simply represent a new or more immature stage in the development of these qualities. Distinguishing pastel or light shades of color from muted colors can at times be difficult, but it is helpful to keep in mind that a muted color is dull in its intensity, and here the dreamer makes specific mention of the beauty and vibrant nature of the colors.

Dream 52:
Testing, Then Treatment

Dreamer: A woman in Ohio

Source: God

Color: Colors

Dream Category: Prophetic dream

Dream: I dreamed that my husband was in a children's hospital for a week, and at the end of the week, one of the medical staff, upon leaving the room, said that we would start the treatment next week. I thought, *What's the treatment?* Then I woke up.

Dreamer's Understanding/Interpretation: I sensed that there would be a treatment for my husband's rare disorder, and that he would get the treatment.

Author's Spirit-Led Interpretation: There is something your husband needs that is coming, but it is not yet here. Although you don't yet know what it is, don't let go of the promise that it is coming.

Impact/Outcome: This dream gave me hope to continue to believe for a treatment for my husband's rare condition, hypophosphastasia. We had been told over the years that we would never see a treatment in his lifetime. Though we did not know it, however, a medicine called Strensiq was just beginning to be developed at the time of my dream in 2009. Most of the trials and research were being done in children's hospitals. In 2016, my husband received treatment with this medicine and he has seen positive results. After being required to use a powered chair 95 percent of the time over the preceding eight years due to soft bones, he is now undergoing physical therapy and is walking with a wheeled walker. It took months to get approval for the medicine, but the dream gave us faith to keep pursuing it.

Primary Metaphor(s):

Children's hospital—a place of healing, but in this case, it also represents healing that is not yet fully developed

Next week—timing, something that is not for today, but is yet to come

Lesson: It is amazing how God can use symbols in dreams in such unique and creative ways. A hospital, by its very nature, is a place for healing, and frequently it will represent a gift or call to a healing ministry or at times a healing vocation. However, in this dream, the meaning shifts just slightly to provide greater confirmation for the dreamer that what the dream promises is real and is in fact for her family. The fact that the dream involved a hospital for children—those whose bodies are not yet fully developed into their adult state—indicates the status of the medicine that was still in development at the time of the dream. In addition, by choosing this metaphor, God was also giving the dreamer a sign by which she could know what treatment the dream was promising. When the dreamer learned that the medication was being researched in children's hospitals, it built confidence to believe that a treatment would soon be available for adults, including her husband, just as the dream had promised.

While some might have concerns that this dream is not from God because it promotes hope in a treatment and a medication instead of in divine healing, the opposite is in fact true. It is important to remember that all knowledge, including medical knowledge, is a gift from God. Regardless of whether healing comes from a miraculous impartation of the Holy Spirit or from the skillful use of medical knowledge, it is still a gift from God. In particular, by giving the dreamer this dream, God also encouraged her (allowing this dream to also be classified as a courage dream) that this natural means of healing was for her husband when she learned about it.

Dream 53:
Streams to Australia

Dreamer: A woman in Australia

Source: God

Color: Colors

Dream Category: Direction dream

Dream: I am walking along the most beautiful beach I've ever seen. The waters are beautiful sea-green; the sand is a dark, golden color with flakes of shiny gold sparkling in the sunlight. The wind is blowing pretty hard, but it's refreshing. My hair is blowing back in the wind, and I'm loving it. I notice the sea foam is thick and luscious. It almost looks like whipped cream. I can't resist, so I bend down and scoop up some on my fingers to taste it. It is sweet and salty at the same time—very nice. In the distance, I can see houses and buildings, but one particular building is right on the water. I know this is where I live. I walk over to the building, and it looks like there is an arboretum on one end. I walk into the back door, and there is a man there conducting experiments. He stands, greets me, and opens a door that leads to a house-type section of the building. As I walk down the hallway, it seems familiar to me, but I cannot figure out why. I look into a room filled with books, and I see a huge Bible on a stand. I see my husband's legs sticking out from underneath the stand. I walk over to him, and he has the Bible in his hands. I ask him what he is doing, and he says that he is studying. I go on down the hallway and open two double doors that lead to a cafeteria-type room with tables and chairs. There are lots of people I know in there. I see John Paul Jackson and many other folks whom I recognize from my church. I assume this is the Streams offices. I am greeted by one of the ladies and led into the room to a table. I sit down and look around the room for quite some time. Then these snakes, scorpions, and other bugs start crawling all over the place. I am a bit freaked out. People begin to flood out of the room. I look up to see John Paul and two other leaders on a stage. I grab a nearby chair and begin to scoot the creeping things out of my way so I can get out the door. I go out the door, closing it behind me, and find myself in an auditorium or a theater-type room. I see my family in a row close to the front. I go down and get in with my family. The lights dim, the curtain opens, and I wake up.

Dreamer's Understanding/Interpretation: I didn't understand this dream until it came to pass.

Author's Spirit-Led Interpretation: There is a move coming that will take you to a new place of peace. Along the way, you have the opportunity to be spiritually fed and grow in relationship with Streams Ministries. Circumstances will help clarify when the time comes to clear the way and for you to move on with your family, for the curtain to open on the next chapter of your destiny.

Impact/Outcome: I had this dream in 2003, at a time when my husband and I were not very good at dream interpretation. However, since that time, we have walked out the elements of the dream and have come to understand it. The beach from my dream turned out to be a very real beach in Middleton, South Australia. We've actually walked on that beach. The house and the cafeteria that I felt were Streams offices related to a time we spent working for Streams Ministries, but at the time of the dream, we had not yet worked there. In 2007, my husband and I went to Australia for a second time and taught a class in Mount Gambier. We were traveling from that class to Melbourne to teach another class and were driving along the great ocean road, getting used to driving on the opposite side of the road and from the opposite side of the car, and talking about how much we loved Mount Gambier (even that we would love to live there if that door ever opened). However, we knew that our employer at Streams, John Paul Jackson, wanted us to move to Melbourne or Adelaide, which were much larger cities.

I was driving, when all of a sudden, my husband shouted for me to turn left. It happened so quickly that I couldn't make the turn and so I took the next left. Then I heard a voice say to look up, and the street name was the same as my own name. I was pretty shaken up by that as we drove down to the beach. We got out of the car and walked along the beach, and I was in awe. This was the beach from my dream. Even the buildings and houses were exactly the same as they had been in my dream. Of course, the Streams building from my dream was not there, but everything else was, including the golden sand with gold flakes (which I later learned was called "mica").

My husband and I walked along the beach in silence, listening for the Holy Spirit to speak. We thought perhaps this was where we were supposed to move. As we left the parking area, we saw a sign that said Middleton, but both of us misread it to say "middle town" and we later learned that Mount Gambier was exactly in the "middle way" between Melbourne and Adelaide. The next day, in Melbourne, while teaching our class, we had six people who had driven up from Mount Gambier. They took us to lunch and told us that they wanted to be our sponsors into the country. After moving to Mount Gambier, we found out that we could not have moved anywhere else in the country and gained residency because we were too old. There was a cutoff for immigration into Australia at the age of forty-five and we were each forty-seven. Mount Gambier had a special immigration policy in place that lifted the age limit to fifty.

As we prepared to move the following August, we learned that some of the same circumstances that had signaled the timing of our move had also resulted in Streams being unable to financially support our move. We knew—because of the dream—that we needed to go anyway. God had known what would happen and He had arranged a plan for us to move to Mount Gambier, exactly as He had shown us in the dream.

Primary Metaphor(s):

Arboretum—a place of growth

Cafeteria—a place to be fed

Snakes, scorpions, and bugs—issues (perhaps demonic attacks) that would cause people to relocate

Chair—authority over the enemy and his plans (see Ephesians 2:6)

Theater curtain opening—the stage is set and it is time for the show to begin

Lesson: Notice how this dream mixes metaphorical symbols with literal images. Such a mixture is a wonderful illustration of why it can be difficult to distinguish the difference between what is a dream and what is a vision, even when using the definition indicated at the beginning of this book (that *visions* are literal, while *dreams* need interpretation). The beach and most of the buildings were quite literal and provided vital confirmation of the geographical location where the dreamer and her family were supposed to move in Australia when the time came. The location was not a place that they had seen before the dream, and thus, it was not something that had arisen from the dreamer's subconscious, but rather it was a divine impartation of information concerning the direction that God was providing. This is just one of the reasons that it is not advisable for those who would interpret dreams to rely upon dream dictionaries as a primary source of understanding symbols. It is essential that those who would interpret dreams rely upon the voice of the Holy Spirit, who, as the Giver of the dream, already knows which images are literal and which are symbolic.

Additionally, this dream illustrates the significance of recognizing that interpretations can come in a multitude of ways, but that the interpretations belong to God (see Genesis 40:8), and that He has the liberty to release those interpretations as He wills. Although the dreamer did not have a mature understanding of dream interpretation, she did work at Streams Ministries for a season (a ministry known for its expertise in biblical dream interpretation), and she still received no direct interpretation to the dream. Instead, God chose to release the interpretation to this dream as the dream came to pass, thus both providing the dreamer with the confidence to be obedient and preventing her from taking pride in knowing the steps of the journey upon which she and her husband were going to be embarking.

Finally, this dream also provided distinct timing, although that timing was veiled until an understanding of the dream interpretation became clear. Though Streams was unable to provide financial support for a move that had been planned, it did not change the timing of the move. Circumstances at Streams Ministries resulted in several people needing to leave. Such circumstances, though perhaps resulting from an attack of the enemy (scorpions, snakes, and bugs that caused people to depart the cafeteria in the dream), were a direct indication of God's timing.

Dream 54:
The Watch Dream

Dreamer: A seven-year-old boy in Virginia

Source: God

Color: Colors

Dream Category: Word of Knowledge/Calling dream

Dream: I was watching a movie with Mommy, Daddy, and my brother. In my dream, they were watching the movie, but I was looking for part of my orange Star Wars BB-8 watch. There was another lady helping me who was wearing glowing white clothes, but I didn't know who she was. I then heard a voice that said, "Look in the closet corner." I opened this closet and saw the rest of my watch. I put the watch back together, put it on, and then I woke up.

Dreamer's Understanding/Interpretation: I talked to my mom and dad and told them my dream. My mom asked, "Did God show you where the watch is yet?" Daddy felt that it was time for me "to watch" (that is, become a watchman).

Author's Spirit-Led Interpretation: God wants to provide all the pieces you need to do something new in your life and help you become a watchman in His Kingdom.

Impact/Outcome: I was happy and excited and knew that God was speaking to me. God loves me and He knows me personally, even down to the watch I wear. I had lost my Star Wars watch, so I went to my room and asked God where the watch was. I looked in the corner of my closet, but it was not there. I felt like I should look in the corner of my bed, under the mattress, and when I did, I found my watch there.

Primary Metaphor(s):

Watch—word play "to watch"; also literal in this case

Woman in glowing white clothes—angel

Closet—hidden

Eight—new beginnings

Lesson: This dream has two very distinct interpretations, and both are completely applicable. The first of these interpretations can be considered a Word of Knowledge dream that provides the dreamer with information that is needed, while the second is more of a calling dream that indicates something about the dreamer's destiny. On the same night that this child dreamed about finding his Star Wars watch, both his brother and his mother also had dreams about watches; however, this was the only one related to the missing watch. This helps to clarify that part of this dream is about a purpose God has both for this boy and for his family—to empower them as intercessors and watchmen in the Kingdom.

While the calling portion of this dream is powerful, it would likely have had only limited impact in the life of a seven-year-old child, while the Word of Knowledge portion of the dream will be remembered for quite some time. Finding the watch provides the dreamer with the needed confidence to recognize that God cares about him personally and to believe he does actually have a purpose in the Kingdom, even at such a young age. Notice that in waking life, the watch was not found in the closet as it was in the dream. This does not detract from the prophetic nature of the dream whatsoever. The closet in the dream could be a place where things are stored or a place (particularly in the life of a child) where things are hidden. Although there are often very literal symbols in a Word of Knowledge dream, this does not mean that there are not times when the symbols need to be interpreted. The dream encourages the dreamer to look for the watch in the corner of a hidden place, but then he remained dependent on the Holy Spirit to hear where that hiding place actually was.

In the end, by helping this child find something he valued that had been missing, God also encouraged him concerning his value in the Kingdom and ensured that he would hear what his parents had to say about his purpose and destiny.

Dream 55:
The Domain Name from Jesus

 *(Use the QR code to hear the dreamer give more details about the dream and its significance. If you do not have access to a QR code reader, the Web site associated with this dream is listed in the INDEX.)*

Dreamer: A woman in Alabama

Source: God

Color: Full colors

Dream Category: Invention dream

Dream: I took a nap and told my husband I would help him when I woke up. In my dream, a man with a gray beard and a blue shirt came up to me and said, "Name it *Tradewind Studios*," then he smiled super big. I woke up.

Dreamer's Understanding/Interpretation: I was to name my business Tradewind Studios.

Author's Spirit-Led Interpretation: This is a direct answer from the Lord. He is revealing to you the name that should be used for your new business.

Impact/Outcome: For one week, my husband and I had been trying to come up with a good name that was available for his new business and its website. The Internet domain name for everything we loved had already been taken or was only available at a price that was beyond our budget.

We must have tried over two hundred names easily already, though my husband felt it was even more than that. It was starting to feel ridiculous. We had been searching for names, when I took a nap and had the dream. After waking, I ran to my husband and said, "Try this name and see if it's taken." I didn't know what the name meant, but I knew the smile from my dream very well. My husband's eyes got huge and he said, "It's available!" This was the first time we had seen those words during our entire search. We went to look up what the name meant and were in awe. It said, a"The prevailing winds of the southern region near the equator." Living in the southern United States, we took this to be related to us. We felt the word *trade* related to our gifts and abilities that would be featured on the site and the word *wind* spoke of the Holy Spirit.

After finding all of this out, we went to purchase the domain name, but it wasn't available anymore. We tried several times to no avail, so we prayed, "God, that's our name! We want it back." We felt so strongly that it would come back to us that we decided not to look up any more names that night. We just tried again the following morning, and we got it. This was the most straightforward dream I have ever had, and it allowed us to save significant time and spend it in quality time together instead of searching for names.

Primary Metaphor(s):

Man—God

Gray beard—wisdom

Blue—revelation

Lesson: This is a great dream that could also be considered a vision due to its straightforward nature. It could also be classified as prophetic, because at its simplest form it is actually a prophetic declaration to the dreamer. While it is not an absolute invention dream, it still fits the category because it provides the information that was needed to create something that the dreamer did not have prior to the dream. In this case, the domain name for a Web site, which (for those unfamiliar with how a Web site is developed) is essential to the creation of the site itself and the Web site cannot be created without it.

This dream also illustrates the need to lay hold of and pursue what God promises, both in dreams and through other means of revelation. When the dreamer paused to look up the meaning of the name, the enemy sought to bring discouragement through giving the appearance that the name was no longer available. Instead of giving in to the discouragement, the dreamer set their heart on the promise that God had made, claimed the dream, and went to sleep with the peace that God would provide what He had promised. By clinging to the promise and pursuing it, instead of falling into a place of loss or regret, the dreamer overcame the enemy's attack and the fulfillment of the dream became even more encouraging.

CONCLUSION

Dreams are an amazing way that God has chosen to speak to His people, yet they have little significance if we fail to value them or even listen to what He is saying through them. To illustrate this point, consider the following. Hundreds, perhaps thousands, of dreamers experienced dreams related to the events surrounding the September 11 attacks against the United States of America. One such dream was experienced by a young woman, who described it as follows:

> *It was the summer of 2001. I had just graduated from high school. I woke up one morning after a night of dreaming, as I often did, but this was different. This dream was burned onto my consciousness and I could not let it go. I told everyone that I thought might hear me out about this dream, seeking opinions or insight. The dream began with me as a first person. I was in a red-skirted suit inside an extremely tall office building, which was shaking. I ran to a group of coworkers and we huddled in a circle to pray. I got up and went to the window and peered up at the building next to me that I knew was as tall as or taller than the building I was in. I*

watched as a jet struck the building and I knew that we were under attack.

This dreamer went on to describe her understanding of the dream as if it was a window into the future and knowing that it meant that life was about to change dramatically. The biggest challenge for this dreamer was what should be done with the dream. While she recognized that the dream was significant and she sought opinions and insight from others, it still seemed after September 11, 2001, that something more should have been done. People all over the world experienced dreams such as this and the corresponding sense that something had been missed.

It is unlikely that by writing this book, peoples' understanding of dreams and what to do with them will suddenly change. However, it is my hope that by sharing these dream stories—these testimonies of how God has changed the lives of real people by speaking to them through dreams—people's understanding of the value and significance of dreams will increase. As the recognition of dreams as one means by which God speaks to His people is restored, and as people begin to seek an understanding of what He is saying through them, the opportunities for dreams both to change individual lives and to impact the course of local, regional, national, and even international events should increase.

REVIEW REQUEST

I hope you have gained some insight about dreams and how important they are by reading this book.

Now that you've read *Dream Stories: Unlocking Your Night Parables*, if you enjoyed it, then please let other readers know. Let's share the knowledge of the importance of dreams and help people everywhere to hear the Lord in new ways.

Dream Stories by Michael B. French

ABOUT THE AUTHOR

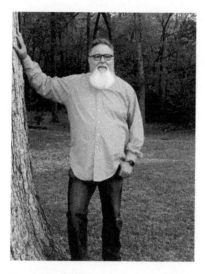

After practicing law for ten years, Michael received his call into full-time Christian ministry. He has passionately ministered all around the globe since then. Michael is the founder of Cahaba Equipping Center, a ministry devoted to training and equipping leaders around the world. Michael is also the founder and president of Patria Ministries (www.patriamin.com), an international association of churches and ministries headquartered in Birmingham, Alabama. Michael and his wife, Elisa, live in Leeds, Alabama. They have four sons: Joshua (wife, Michelle), Caleb, Jacob, and Noah.

www.michaelbfrench.com

Authors' Acknowledgments

I want to first make clear that without the mentoring and training of my spiritual father, John Paul Jackson, my understanding of dreams and the biblical method of interpretation would have remained almost nonexistent. John Paul's teaching and the resources available from Streams Ministries are of tremendous importance to the Body of Christ, and those specifically acknowledged here are only a fraction of what is available.

The Art of Hearing God, is a course about learning to hear God's voice for yourself. This course was authored and developed by John Paul Jackson, and it is available through Streams Ministries both online (see www.streamsministries.com/Classroom) and for groups via a live teacher certified by Streams Ministries.

Understanding Dreams and Visions is a course that lays the foundation for biblical dream interpretation. Also authored and developed by John Paul Jackson, this course can be taken in an online format, taught by John Paul himself (see www.streamsministries.com/Classroom) or for groups via a live teacher certified by Streams Ministries.

Advanced Workshop in Dreams and Visions is a more advanced course on biblical dream interpretation, and it can be taken in an online format, taught by John Paul Jackson (see www.streamsministries.com/Classroom) or for groups via a live teacher certified by Streams Ministries.

Other books, teaching CDs, and resources on biblical dream interpretation are also available from Streams Ministries via their online store at www.streamsministries.com/store.

Other Books
by Michael French

Fresh Bread:
Finding Your Daily Portion in the Lord's Prayer

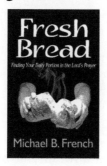

Our Lord, the Great Baker, prepares a special loaf of bread for us each day to sustain us for that day's specific events. Through the Lord's Prayer, He extends an invitation to sit at His table and allow Him to break open this fresh bread for us. More than simply a book on the Lord's Prayer, *Fresh Bread* explains this ancient prayer and shows how it unlocks divine destiny and empowers us to become all that we were created to be. It's time to find your daily portion! And once you do, you'll never again be satisfied with anything less than the fresh bread prepared daily by the Lord especially for you.

Remedy:
Freedom Through Deliverance

2014 Readers' Favorite Bronze Award
in Christian Biblical Counseling

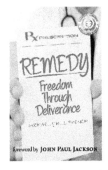

Deliverance ministry is a touchy subject. Just mention the word *deliverance*, and many people conjure up images of *The Exorcist* and other media stereotypes. At a time when the world is confused about deliverance, *Remedy* offers insights on the true authority that Christ intends every believer to walk in. Written by renowned experts Michael and Bill French, this book covers foundational elements and application of deliverance ministry and includes real-life experiences over their sixty-plus combined years of ministry. The foreword by John Paul Jackson emphasizes the spiritual authority that believers wield in the war raging in people's lives.

The Elisha Way:
Preparing for the Double Portion

2013 Readers' Favorite Bronze Award in Christian Living

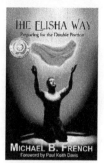

The generation today has the opportunity to experience the power and presence of God in a way that no other generation before them has. They are an Elisha generation on the brink of taking up their mantle and walking in a double anointing.

Dream Stories by Michael B. French

Dedication

This book is dedicated to the men and women who make up Streams Ministries. This ministry and all those associated with it have created an atmosphere that has allowed my gifts to flourish and the truths that God has planted in my life to take root and grow.

Streams Ministries was founded by John Paul Jackson, who, throughout his lifetime, created an environment that emphasized character over giftedness and encouraged people to see the awe of God restored in the earth. John Paul and the courses he developed drew me into the realm of biblical dream interpretation and helped me to see this amazing gift that much of the Body of Christ had overlooked for generations. Dianne Jackson, his wife, faithfully supported her husband, and her enduring friendship with my family helps to keep us grounded in the place where our gifts can continue to grow. Mike and Amanda Wise and the diverse staff that Streams has had over the years (too numerous to mention by name) have been both great friends and powerful encouragers as we have taken this journey into the world of dream interpretation. Finally, the Streams Training Center leaders and teachers, such as Recie Saunders, John Thomas (now the president of Streams Ministries), Scott Evelyn, Tony and Dwee Cooke, Kristi Graner, and many, many more who took this journey with us have provided the iron against which my iron could be sharpened. This book would not have been possible without all of these amazing individuals who made up and continue to make up what is Streams Ministries.

INDEX OF DREAMS

Use the QR code to hear the dreamer give more details about the dream and its significance. If you do not have access to a QR code reader, use the Website address.

www.MyDreamStories.com

Dream 2: A Visit from the Surgeon

http://mydreamstories.com/Dreams/AVisitFromTheSurgeon.html

Dream 3: A Father's Forgiveness

http://mydreamstories.com/Dreams/AFathersForgiveness.html

Dream 4: Battle for My Son

http://mydreamstories.com/Dreams/BattleForMySon.html

Dream 6: Cutting My Tongue Out

http://mydreamstories.com/Dreams/CuttingMyTongueOut.html

Dream 11: John Paul Jackson Takes a Bite of Eggs

http://www.mydreamstories.com/john-paul-jackson-takes-a-bite-of-e

Dream 12: Airplane Crash into Ocean

http://mydreamstories.com/Dreams/AirplaneCrashIntoOcean.html

Dream 14: I'm in Charge Here!

http://mydreamstories.com/Dreams/ImInChargeHere.html

Dream 15: Will I Sink?

http://mydreamstories.com/Dreams/WillISink.html

Dream 19: Don't Give Up

http://mydreamstories.com/Dreams/DontGiveUp.html

Dream 20: Destiny Choice

http://mydreamstories.com/Dreams/DestinyChoice.html

Dream 23: Computer Spider

http://mydreamstories.com/Dreams/ComputerSpider.html

Dream 24: Herobrine in the Basement

http://mydreamstories.com/Dreams/HerobrineInTheBasement.html

Dream 31: Little Blind Girl

http://mydreamstories.com/Dreams/LittleBlindGirl.html

Dream 32: Get That Mole Checked

http://mydreamstories.com/Dreams/GetThatMoleChecked.html

Dream 40: A Dream Come True

http://mydreamstories.com/Dreams/ADreamComeTrue.html

Dream 42: The Truth About My Father and My Grief

http://www.mydreamstories.com/truth-about-my-father

Dream 48: Minefield

http://mydreamstories.com/Dreams/MineField.html

Dream 50: 1987 Market Crash

http://www.mydreamstories.com/market-crash

Dream 55: The Domain Name from Jesus

www.mydreamstories.com/domain-name-from-jesus

REFERENCES

[1] Madison Park. "90 Percent of U.S. Bills Carry Traces of Cocaine." 17 August 2009. CNN. Web. 21 July 2015. <http://www.cnn.com/2009/HEALTH/08/14/cocaine.traces.money/>

[2] "The Martyrdom of Polycarp." Ed. Dan Graves. Trans. J.B. Lightfoot. Comp. Stephen Tomkins. n.d. <https://www.christianhistoryinstitute.org/study/module/polycarp/>.

[3] John Boruff. "Tertullian on Dreams." 20 April 2014. WesleyGospel.com. Web. 22 July 2015.

[4] Christian History Institute. "Persecution in Early Church: Did You Know?" *Christian History* 1990: 10. <https://www.christianhistoryinstitute.org/uploaded/50cf7cb17495c9.82992192.pdf>.

[5] Synesius of Cyrene. *De Insomniis (On Dreams)* by Saint Synesios. Trans. Isaac Myer. Philadelphia: Harvard College Library, 1888.

[6] Aquinas, *Summa Theologica* II-II, Q. 95, Art. 6

[7] Thomas Aquinas. "*Summa Theologica.*" Treatise on the Cardinal Virtues. Vol. Question 95. Of Superstition in Divinations. n.d. Print.

[8] A&E Television Networks. "St. Thomas Aquinas." 2015. Bio. Web. 23 July 2015.

[9] Craig Cross. *The Beatles: Day-by-Day, Song-by-Song, Record-by-Record.* Lincoln: iUniverse, Inc., 2005. Print.

[10] Geoff Boucher. "Inception Breaks into Dreams." 4 April 2010. *Los Angeles Times.* Web. 23 July2015 2015.

[11] Trinitarius. "An Opinion on Dreams. *Burton's Gentleman's Magazine* (August 1839): 105. Print.

[12] George K. York III, MD. "Otto Loewi: Dream Inspires Nobel-Winning Experiment on Neurotransmission." 25 September 2014. *Neurology Today.* Web. 23 July 2015.

[13] Ward Hill Lamon. *Recollections of Abraham Lincoln 1847-1865.* Lincoln: University of Nebraska Press, 1994. Print.

[14] Lord Byron. "The Dream." *The World's Best Poetry,* edited by Bliss Carman, et al Philadelphia: John D. Morris & Co., 1904; Bartleby.com, 2012. http://www.bartleby.com/360/3/34.html

[15] John H. Lienhard. *Engines of Our Ingenuity.* 2003. Web. 23 July 2015.

[16] A'Lelia Perry Bundles. *Madam C.J. Walker: Entrepreneur.* New York: Chelsea House Publishers, 1991. Print.

[17] S.T. Coleridge, Esq. Christabel, &c. Third Edition. St. James: William Bulmer and Co., 1816. Print. 24 July 2015. <http://special.lib.gla.ac.uk/teach/romanticism/kublaprefl.html>.

[18] Jonathan Jones. "Is it patriotic? Subversive? Both? Jonathan Jones on how Jasper Johns made a provocative masterpiece out of the American flag." 22 April 2003. *The Guardian.* Web. 24 July 2015. <http://www.theguardian.com/artanddesign/2003/apr/22/artsfeatur es>.

[19] BBC News. "Five Dream Discoveries." 10 June 2009. http://news.bbc.co.uk/go/pr/fr/- /2/hi/uk_news/magazine/8092029.stm. Web. 14 August 2015.

[20] NBC. The Voice. 1 March 2016. 22 March 2016. <http://www.nbc.com/the-voice/episode-guide/season-10/the-blind- auditions-premiere-part-2/1002>.

[21] NBC. The Voice. 1 March 2016. 22 March 2016. <http://www.nbc.com/the-voice/episode-guide/season-10/the-blind- auditions-premiere-part-2/1002>.

[22] Please see Author's Acknowledgments at the end of this book for more information on this course

[23] Wise, Michael. *The 20 Categories of Dreams: Understanding the Various Ways God Speaks Through Dreams.* Dallas: Streams Ministries International, 2015. Print

[24] This dream was presented to a minister on a mission trip to Poland with John Paul Jackson in 2004. The dream and interpretation is presented here as recounted by the ministry team. The interpreter was seated in a pub with a group of young people anxious to learn about dreams when two drunk men entered the pub and became quite obnoxious. One of the young people stood up and told the men that they were trying to visit with the American minister and they were being disturbed by the men's behavior. The two men continued to disrupt the visit. The minister felt the Lord's prompting to ask if the one of the men had experienced a dream the previous night. This dream was his response.

CPSIA information can be obtained
at www.ICGtesting.com
Printed in the USA
LVHW090202020219
606149LV00001B/35/P

9 781937 331726